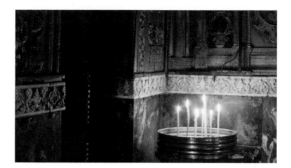

AROMATIC CANDLES

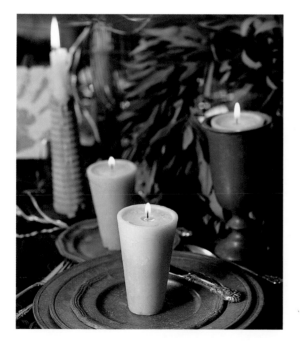

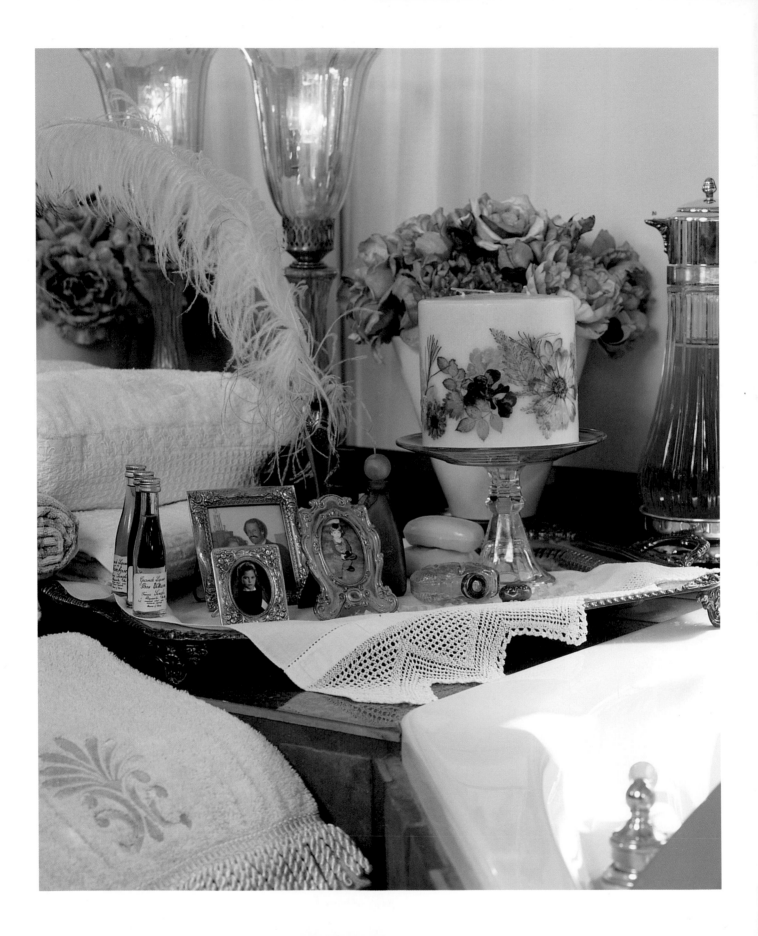

AROMATIC CANDLES

Rosevita Warda

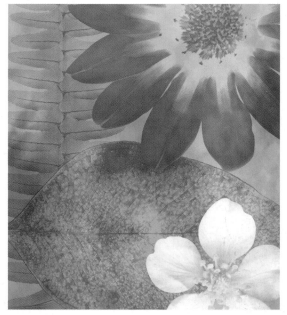

Sterling Publishing Co., Inc. New York
A Sterling/Chapelle Book

Chapelle Ltd.

Owner:
Jo Packham

Editor:
Kristi C. Torsak

Staff:
Areta Bingham, Kass Burchett,
Jill Dahlberg, Marilyn Goff,
Holly Hollingsworth, Susan Jorgensen,
Barbara Milburn, Linda Orton,
Karmen Quinney, Cindy Stoeckl,
Kim Taylor, Sara Toliver, Desirée Wybrow

Photographers:
Kevin Dilley for Hazen Imaging Inc.,
Scot Zimmerman Photography,
Luciana Pampolone

Photodisc, Inc. Images (© 1992, 1993, 1995, 1996, 1999, 2000)
Corbis Corporation Images (© 1998, 2001)
Artville, LLC Images (© 1997)

Library of Congress Cataloging-in-Publication Data
Warda, Rosevita.
    Aromatic candles / Rosevita Warda.
        p. cm.
    Includes index.
ISBN 0-8069-8735-9
1. Candlemaking. 2. Essences and essential oils.
3. Aromatherapy I. Title

TT896.5 . W35 2001
745.593'32--dc21

2001034854

10 9 8 7 6 5 4 3 2 1
Published by Sterling Publishing Company, Inc.,
387 Park Avenue South, New York, NY 10016
© 2001 by Rosevita Warda
Distributed in Canada by Sterling Publishing
c/o Canadian Manda Group, One Atlantic Avenue, Suite 105
Toronto, Ontario, Canada M6K 3E7
Distributed in Great Britain and Europe by Cassell PLC
Wellington House, 125 Strand, London WC2R 0BB, England
Distributed in Australia by Capricorn Link (Australia) Pty Ltd.
P.O. Box 704, Windsor, NSW 2756, Australia
Printed in China
All Rights Reserved
Sterling ISBN 0-8069-8735-9

If you have any questions or comments, please contact:

Chapelle Ltd., Inc.
P. O. Box 9252
Ogden, UT 84409
(801) 621-2777 FAX (801) 621-2788
e-mail: Chapelle@chapelleltd.com
website: www.chapelleltd.com

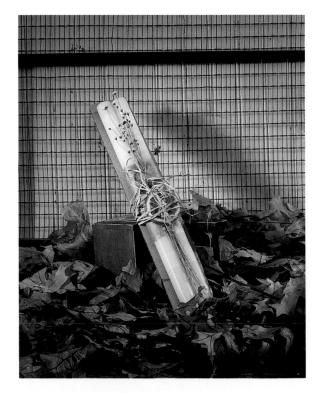

FROM THE AUTHOR

My childhood years were spent in Frankfurt, Germany. From there, I went on to work as a journalist, crafts person, organic gardener/farmer, candlemaker and soapmaker, mother, and businesswoman. I have lived in various corners of the world and have enjoyed the many different cultures and environments that I have encountered. Through these experiences, I have learned to appreciate genuine beauty—and to value the treasures nature provides to support happiness and well being.

"Delight Company," my first enterprise in the U.S., started out offering soaps, candles, and aromatherapy products over the Internet (www.delightcompany.com). Delight Company has since merged with AromaLand in Santa Fe, New Mexico, where I currently work as Vice President of Sales and Marketing. I am proud to be a part of a company that is strongly committed to quality.

Learning the secrets of aromatherapy is a valuable source of joy for me. The sensations are thrilling; these precious plant essences affect me on many different levels. It is also enticing to know that there is always much more to be learned and experienced! I strongly believe that only nature can take our lives back to their roots and to natural well being.

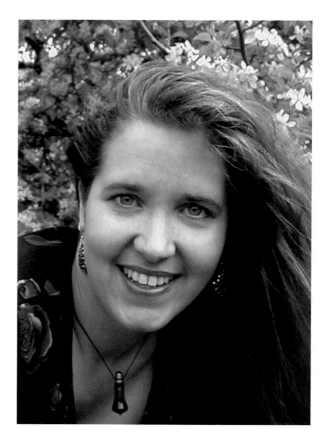

To my daughter Tiamat, and friends and family who nurtured me along my way.

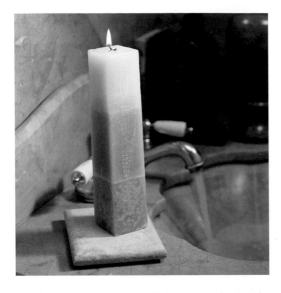

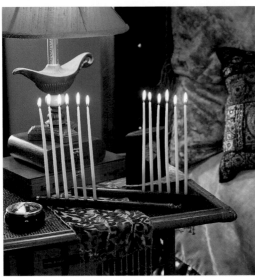

TABLE
OF
CONTENTS

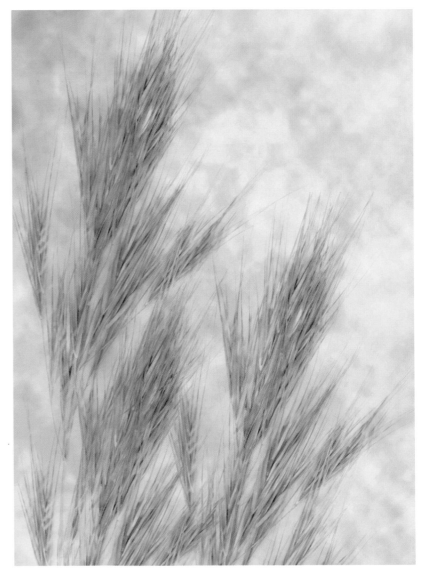

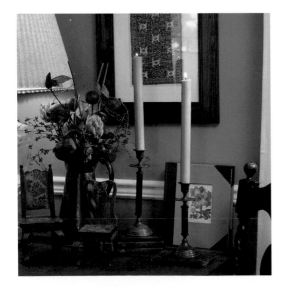

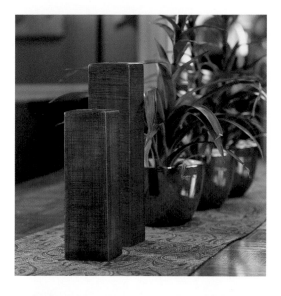

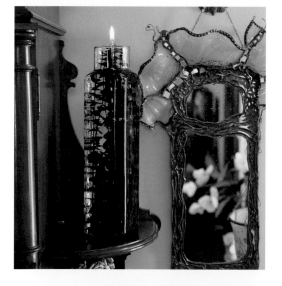

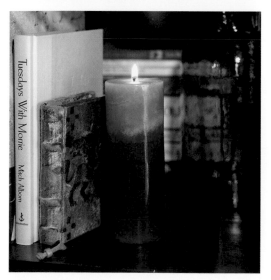

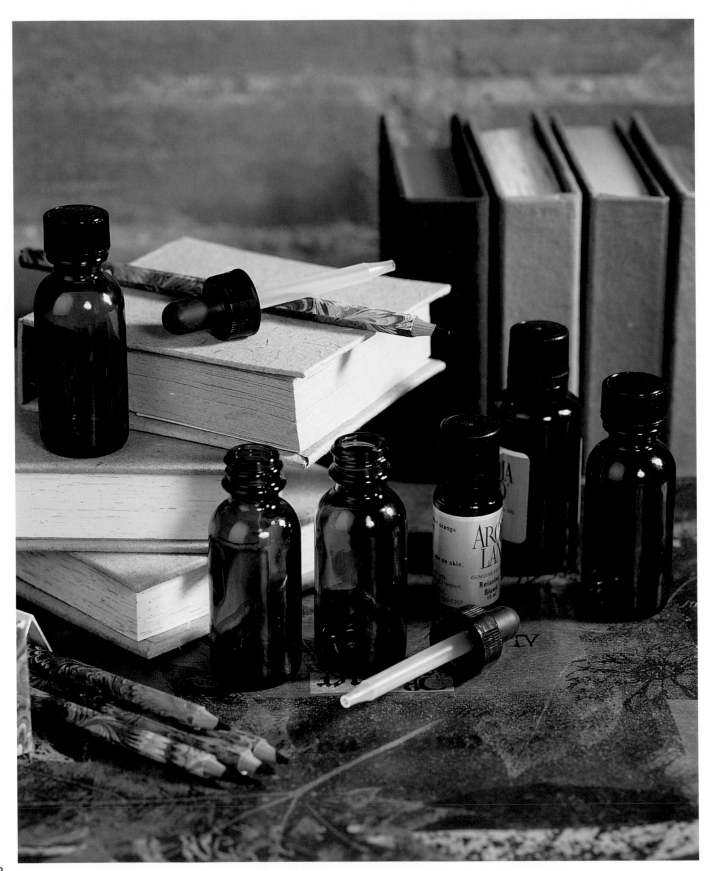

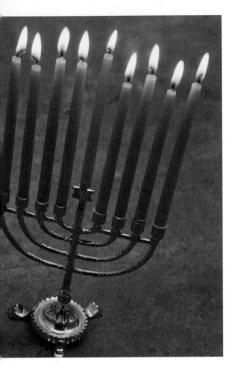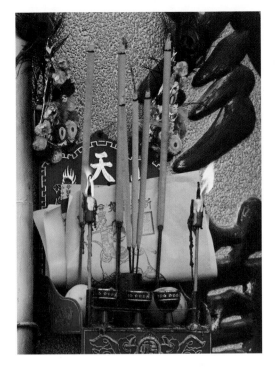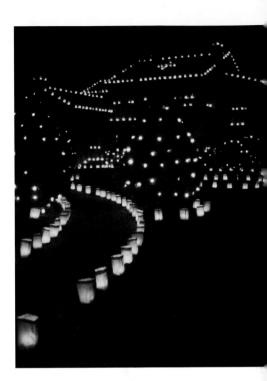

INTRODUCTION

Scenting candles with essential oils is a very satisfying and rewarding craft. Aromatherapy, through handmade candles, enhances mood as well as adding a little ceremony to your daily life. Since mankind has taken possession of fire, we have used it in powerful rituals to reconcile and soothe body, soul, and mind.

Fire fascinates us—soft at times and wild at other times. Humans, throughout time, have used the power of fire to add depth and drama to ceremonies and celebrations. Candlelight can turn eating into dining, resting into meditation, and prayer into devotion. *Aromatic Candles* takes it one step further by combining visual beauty with the experience of scents derived directly from nature. Throughout time and cultures, scent has been used to enhance moods and spiritual experiences. Of all our senses, the sense of smell is probably the closest to the soul. Aromas are directly transmitted to the limbic system—part of the brain where memory, subconscious knowledge, and our basic instincts reside. Because the olfactory nerves in the nose are a direct extension of the brain's limbic system, recognition of scent is relayed immediately and influences our emotions directly, without control or censorship by mind or reason. Scent is the only sense that works immediately, while taste, sound, sight, and touch are processed by the intellect. That is why the natural aromas used in genuine aromatherapy can be such powerful enhancements to our well being.

This book is intended for those of you who desire to be candle poets and scent artists, in hopes that it will empower you to create a unique expression of yourself. You will find that creating a handmade candle with essential oil blends is a special act and has significant value—given as a gift or burned in your own space.

A Few Important Words About Aromatherapy and Essential Oils

Essential oils are the pure essences of healing and aromatic plants. They are the very soul of the plant, a precious extraction, and a true gift from nature. Genuine aromatherapy uses pure essential oils to enhance physical, emotional, and spiritual well being.

The terms "essential oil" and "genuine aromatherapy" imply that the source of the aroma must be 100% natural. If you are looking for therapeutic- and well-being-related effects, there is no alternative to "the real thing."

The majority of the manufacturers of aromatherapy and aromatic candles ignore this fact—calling "aromatherapy" any scent that smells like an essential oil. The terminology has not yet been legally defined, so the consumer is faced with the challenge to distinguish between the authentic and the imitation.

Pure essences are more expensive than the imitations, since it often requires hundreds of pounds of plant matter to extract even a tiny amount, such as an ounce, of essential oil. Additionally, essential oils require a little more care in their storage than do chemically produced fragrances.

Your Nose Knows

Why the concern about the use of a synthetic fragrance that is cheaper and easier to store? Synthetics may be close in scent to an essential oil; however, once you have been introduced to the authentic, natural essences, nothing else will do. Synthetics are artificially produced and occasionally contain ingredients that are suspected to be carcinogen and responsible for various allergic reactions, and

are toxic or reactive to the skin. Additionally, if you are looking to enhance your life with aromatic candles, do not settle for less than 100% pure essential oils. A pure aromatherapy candle is a very unique and precious object, well worth the effort and expense.

Even though the term "essential oil" should describe oil that is 100% natural essence, it is not uncommon for chemical/essential oil fragrance blends or essential oil blended with another "base" oil to be labeled "essential oil." You can use the following information to make certain that you are purchasing 100% natural essence oil:

• Purchase oils from companies that have an established reputation in the aromatherapy field.

• Read the essential oil label. Does it ensure purity? Does it state the botanical name, country of origin, form of extraction, and how the plant was cultivated?

• If the essential oil supplier offers scents such as rain, lily of the valley, and raspberry, be wary. The manufacturer may value synthetic fragrances as comparable substitutes for the real thing.

• Essential oils come in various grades and varieties, so you will need to sniff it out, "literally." Lavender oil, for example, can vary greatly in quality and scent, depending on plant origin, distiller's expertise, and the quality of storage.

• Essential oils may be sold in dilution with natural base oil, since they are overly strong in their pure form, which is fine if they are labeled as such. If you have any questions as to whether or not the essential oil you purchase is at full strength, try placing a drop of oil on a piece of paper and allow it to completely evaporate. The remaining stain should not look like an oily mark, which indicates that the essential oil was stretched with a vegetable oil.

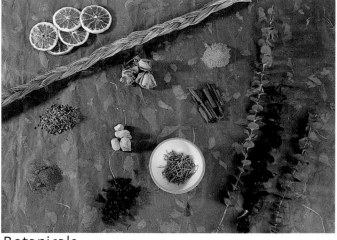
Botanicals

Most scents will fall into one of the following categories:

- Camphorous: pungent, sharp scent—e.g. cajeput, eucalyptus, pine, tea tree

- Citrus: fresh, clean scent—e.g. grapefruit, lemon, lime, mandarin orange, orange, petitgrain

- Floral: flowery scent—e.g. jasmine, lavender, neroli, rose

- Herbal: intense and herbaceous scent—e.g. basil, marjoram, rosemary, sage

- Minty: cool, fresh scent—e.g. peppermint, spearmint

- Resinous: gums or resins scent—e.g. benzoin, elemi, frankincense, myrrh

- Spicy: piquant, sharp scent—e.g. black pepper, cardamom, cinnamon, clove, nutmeg

- Woodsy: freshly cut wood scent—e.g. cedar, cypress, sandalwood

Some scents may be a combination of more than one category, so you may find yourself describing a scent as a combination rather than one type.

Scent Notes

In an analogy to music, perfumers divide essential oil scents into notes:

- Top (head) notes smell light, fresh, and airy. This is normally the first scent you will notice, but this scent also dissipates quickly.

- Middle (heart) notes are more rooted than the top notes, but not extremely heavy in fragrance. These notes form the body of your blend.

- Base notes are heavier and longer lasting, therefore they are dominant after the top and middle notes have evaporated. They may be described as "rich" and they "ground" the blend.

When balancing a blend, the tendency is to incorporate all three types of oil, which should result in a well-layered blend. Keep in mind that the oil blend will merge and alter as it matures. If you are not certain about a blend, allow it to age for a day or two and smell it again—you may be pleasantly surprised!

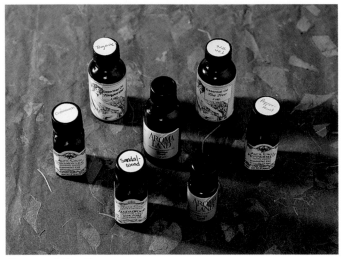
Essential oils

Blending Essential Oils

You need not be an expert to create your own beautifully scented blends, nor do you need recipes—although they tend to be useful in the beginning. All you need to know is what you like and enjoy, and what will work for you.

Treat yourself to an assorted selection of oils. Smell the oils, either passing the bottle directly below your nose, or by putting a few drops on a blotter paper or on unscented tissue. Then sit back and observe the feelings and images the single oil generates. Do you perceive them as calming, energizing, grounding, or sensual? Become acquainted with the individual oils by using them until you become familiar with the various dimensions and qualities that pure essential oils carry.

Making a blend will be like inviting your friends to a party. Your sense of smell will likely go into overload after a few minutes, so take a break or smell some roasted coffee beans. One of the beautiful aspects of making your own blends is that there will always be room for your knowledge and experience to expand. An unlimited bounty of olfactory adventure awaits you!

When blending essential oils you will need a clean glass bottle and separate droppers for each essential oil. Note: Make certain that you remember to use the correct cap and dropper for each oil, so you will not spoil the oils by mixing up the lids.

The following steps will aid you in the blending process:

1. Select the essential oils you would like to blend. Note: There are no rules about how many oils should be in a blend; however, for the beginner, 3–4 oils are recommended.

2. Place an equal number of drops of each oil in the glass bottle.

3. Shake the bottle and test your results.

4. Introduce additional drops of oil a few at a time until you achieve the desired effect.

Always keep detailed notes of the following:

• Essential oils used and the number of drops of each oil

• The therapeutic or personal reasons for the selected oils

• Your perception of the blend, when freshly blended and after maturing

• How the blend performs in candles of different sizes and wicking

It is requisite to take "note keeping" seriously as there is nothing more annoying and frustrating than to create your personal masterpiece, only to realize that you do not remember what you did. Keep a blending journal or notebook where all blends are noted and organized.

Scenting candles with essential oils requires a little more effort and expense than ordinary candlemaking. Essential oils show different characteristics when added to wax and can change from batch to batch. Additionally, there is no guarantee that the scent of the blend that you are using will be the same when the finished candle is burned. Candles made with essential oils may sputter, burn unevenly, or occasionally flare up. It is always a good idea to pour a few "test candles," such as votive size, and burn them down before using a blend in an elaborate and time-intensive candle project. Always keep in mind that a candle should never be left burning unattended—this is particularly important with an aromatherapy candle. The higher the concentration of oils used, the more important it is for one to test and carefully observe the candle as it burns.

The Essential Oils Chart on page 14–15, which was organized with the help of other candlemakers, will assist you in creating your own essential oil blends.

Essential Oils Tips

• Store essential oils and blends in dark glass bottles and in a cool, dark place.

• Always label oils and blends clearly. When labeling blends, be specific. If there is insufficient room on bottle for labeling, try numbering the blend with a corresponding number in your blend notebook.

• Avoid storing your oils with rubber eye dropper tops since the oils may turn the rubber to gum, which will ruin the essential oils.

• Always pay special attention to any safety information listed on the essential oil label. Some essential oils should not be used during pregnancy or with other medical conditions. This primarily applies to topical usage or if ingested, but something that you should be aware of.

Substituting Essential Oils

If you are looking for a therapeutic substitution, try one of the essential oils listed at the beginning of the chapter in conjunction with information from the Essential Oils Chart to help you determine a pleasing blend with the similar therapeutic values. However, if you would like to substitute oils with similar scents while keeping in mind that the therapeutic benefits may vary with the substituted scent, you could try the following:

Oil	Substitution
Vanilla	Benzoin (or Peru Balsam)
Bergamot	Grapefruit
Chamomile	Lavender
Cinnamon	Clove
Jasmine	Ylang-ylang
Lemon	Grapefruit
Neroli	Jasmine (or Ylang-ylang)
Peppermint	Spearmint
Tangerine	Sweet orange

ESSENTIAL OILS CHART

	Basil	Bergamot	Black Pepper	Cardamom	Cedarwood	Chamomile	Cinnamon	Citronella	Clary Sage	Clove	Coriander	Cypress	Eucalyptus	Frankincense	Geranium	Ginger	Grapefruit	Jasmine	Juniper Berry	Lavender	Lemon	Lemongrass
1 Basil		G												G								
2 Bergamot $	F		F	F	H	F	F	H	F					F	F			F	F	F	F	
3 Black Pepper																						
4 Cardamom			S			H			H					S			S					
5 Cedarwood		W		W		W	W							W	W				W	W		W
6 Chamomile $$							F						EX									
7 Cinnamon			S	S					H					S								
8 Citronella									H										H	H		
9 Clary Sage	H	G			G	H	G				G				G		G				H	G
10 Clove			H	S			H							S								
11 Coriander		S	S						G					S		H	S					
12 Cypress		W			H						S				W		W	S				
13 Eucalyptus					H			H												H		
14 Frankincense $	EA	EA		EA	EA		EA		EA		EA				EA					EA		
15 Geranium	EX	EX		EX	EX				EX							EX	H		EX	EX	EX	EX
16 Ginger		S	S						S	H				S								
17 Grapefruit		F	F	F	F	F						F	F		F					F	F	H
18 Jasmine $$$			EX	EX	EX				EX	EX										EX	EX	
19 Juniper Berry		S	S	S			S	S	G	H				S							S	
20 Lavender		G	G	G	H	G		H			G	G	G		G		G		G			G
21 Lemon		F		F		F	F					F	F		F	F	F			F		
22 Lemongrass									H										H	H		
23 Lime		F		F		F	F					F	F		F	F				F	H	
24 Mandarin		H	F	F		F	F			F	F	F			F	H	F			F	F	
25 Marjoram				S																S		
26 Neroli $$$	EX	EX		EX	EX									EX	EX	EX	H			EX	EX	
27 Nutmeg			S			H			H					S								
28 Orange		H	F	F		F	F			F	F				F	H	F			F	F	
29 Patchouli														EA	EA							
30 Peppermint	H																			G	H	
31 Petitgrain										W												
32 Pine										W	S	H							H			
33 Rose $$$			EX	EX	EX	EX								EX	EX			H		EX	EX	
34 Rosemary	G	G		H												G	G					
35 Sandalwood $$			W								W	W			W				W	W	W	W
36 Vanilla $$										EA												
37 Vetiver $									EA					EA	EA							
38 Ylang-ylang			EX	EX	EX	EX													EX		EX	EX

#	Lime	Mandarin Orange	Marjoram	Neroli	Nutmeg	Orange	Patchouli	Peppermint	Petitgrain	Pine	Rose	Rosemary	Sandalwood	Vanilla	Vetiver	Ylang-ylang
1						G					H					
2	F	H	F	F	F	H	F	F	F	F	F	F	F	F		F
3						S					S		S			
4		S				S					S					
5			W			W	W			H	W					W
6			G								G					
7		S			H	S						S		S		
8					H										H	
9	G				G	G	G		G			G			G	
10		S			H	S	S		S	S		S	S			
11		S		S		S					S					
12																
13			F				G	F			H					
14		EA				EA					EA	EA	H			EA
15			H			EX	EX		EX		H		EX		EX	EX
16		S				S	S				S				S	
17	H	F		F	F	H										F
18			H			EX			EX		EX		EX		EX	EX
19		S				S				H		S	S			
20	G		G	G	G	G	G	G	G	G	G	G			G	
21	H	F		F	F	F	F	F	F	F	F	F		F		F
22			H												H	
23		F		F	F	F								F	F	F
24	F			F	F	H					F				F	F
25								S			S					S
26	EX	EX				S	EX		H		H	EX	EX	EX	EX	
27		S				S										
28	F	H		F	F						F		F		F	F
29													H		H	
30			F								H					
31											W					
32											W					
33			EX	EX	EX	EX						EX	EX	EX	EX	
34	G		G		G		H	G	G							
35					W	W					W		W	W	W	
36										S						
37					H								H	EA		EA
38	EX	EX	EX	EX		EX					EX		EX	EX	EX	

Different Ways to Bring Aromatherapy and Candles into Your Life

Purchased aromatic candles can save some of the trouble that may befall a novice candlemaker, since the manufacturer has worked out some of the burning problems. The purchased candles can be used and decorated as desired—a timesaving alternative to beginning from scratch.

Combine candles with additional aromatherapy scenting sources, such as adding an aroma lamp or other diffuser with essential oils to your candle setting. Combining these aromatherapy sources can be an enjoyable experience.

Essential Oils Chart Legend

This legend will help when determining which oils to blend. There are over 300 different commercially produced essential oils today. The thirty-eight essential oils that are on the chart are the most popular and are more readily available. Keep in mind that these are only recommendations and that you can be more adventurous and rely on your sense of smell for what you like.

EA	Make the scent earthier
EX	Make the scent more exotic
F	Freshen the scent
G	Make the scent more herbal
H	Heighten the scent
S	Make the scent spicier
W	Make the scent woodier

Some of the essential oils, marked with $, $$, and $$$ signs, are expensive and because of this, you may choose to use these oils in a diffuser or aroma lamp, rather than crafted into a candle.

Candlemaking

A few supplies and materials are needed for candlemaking and the majority of them can be easily purchased at the local craft store or found around the house. The essential oils may be purchased at the local health food or aromatherapy store, or mail-ordered through a reputable company. Mail-order or the internet will generally be the most economical way to purchase essential oils, although the local health food store or aromatherapy shop may be more convenient.

The following tools and supplies will be necessary for creating candles:

- Candle dye
- Candle molds
- Candle or candy thermometer
- Candle wax
- Candle wick tabs
- Candle wicks
- Double boiler
- Essential oils
- Kitchen scale
- Metal pouring pot
- Mold release
- Mold sealer
- Wax additives

Candle Waxes

If you are making aromatic candles, keep in mind that the softer the wax, the more fragrant the candle seems. Soft wax does not seal its surface as tightly as hard wax does, so it allows the scent to permeate the atmosphere around it. However, soft wax is more appropriate for container candles—tapers or free-standing candles would lose their shape and melt into a pool of wax.

Most manufacturers of candlemaking supplies offer wax compounds that are designed specifically for containers, molds, tapers, etc. This takes some of the guesswork out of trying to determine which additives are necessary for the style of candle that you are making.

Natural Waxes

- Beeswax is highly regarded among candlemakers because it burns beautifully with its own nurturing aroma. Beeswax is stickier than other waxes and requires a slightly larger sized wick. This may also cause problems when releasing a candle containing a high percentage of beeswax from the mold.

Beeswax works best when used in a container, dipped tapers, and rolled candles. Beeswax has a higher melting point (146°F) than most other waxes. It works well when mixed with lower melting-point waxes and used in container candles. Pure beeswax candles will burn directly down the center of the container, leaving much unburned wax on the container walls. Beeswax is available in its natural color or a bleached white and is the most expensive of the waxes. Colored beeswax is also available, but may be a little more difficult to find. If your sheets of beeswax form a dusty-looking film on the surface, remove it by slightly warming the wax surface with a hair dryer.

- Vegetable-based waxes are available and made from different bases. Some are formulated from soybeans, jojoba beans, palm wax, and other vegetable bases. The majority of these waxes are made for container candles rather than pillars or tapers. They burn clean and are long lasting. These waxes may be more diffi-

Continued on page 20.

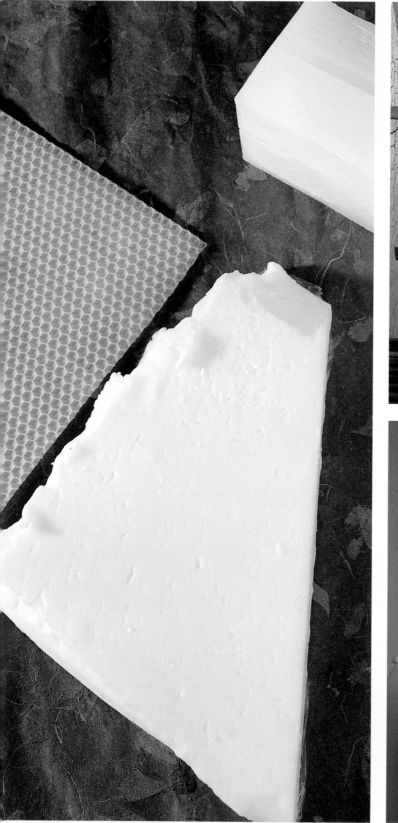

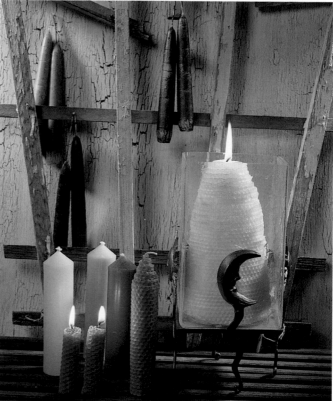

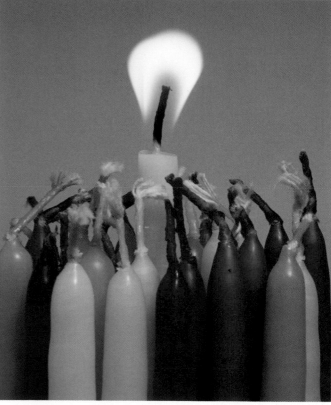

Various candle waxes

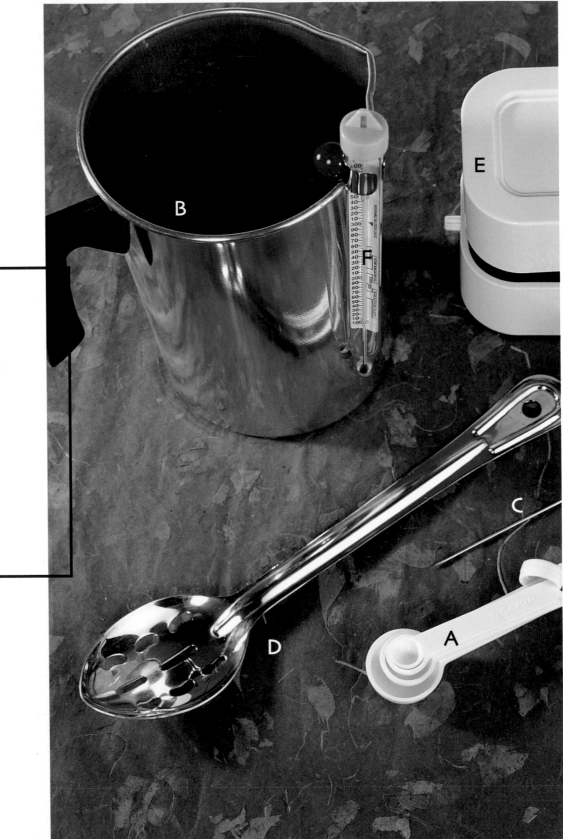

A. Measuring
   spoons

B. Metal pouring
   pot

C. Metal skewer

D. Metal spoon

E. Kitchen scale

F. Thermometer

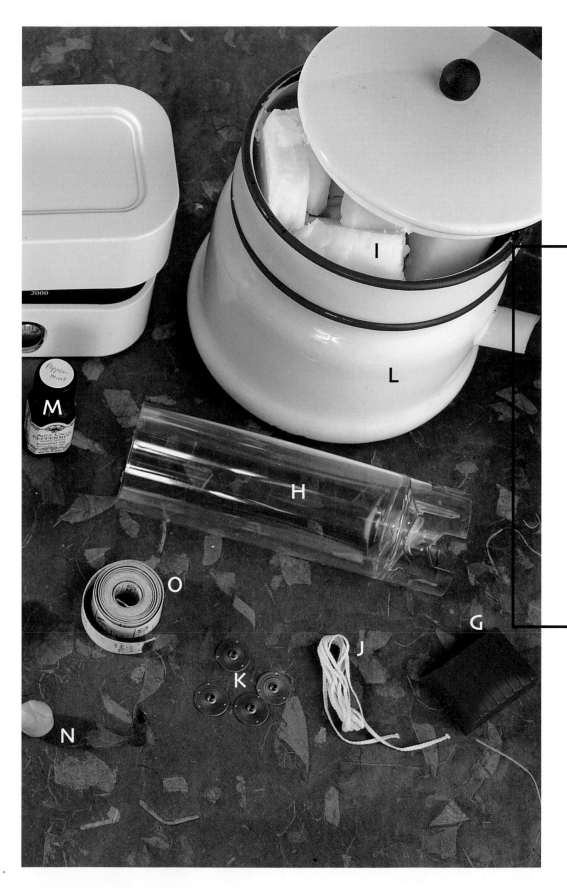

G. Candle dye

H. Candle mold

I. Candle wax

J. Candle wick

K. Candle wick tabs

L. Double boiler

M. Essential oil

N. Mold sealer

O. Tape Measure

Continued from page 16.

cult to find at the local craft store; however, numerous requests by the consumer may help to make them more available in the marketplace. They are also available through mail-order and the internet.

• Bayberry wax is obtained by boiling berries from the bayberry bush. The wax is a sage-green color with a spicy aroma and an equally spicy price. The majority of candles labeled bayberry consist of fragrance added to a regular wax base. When ordering or purchasing bayberry wax, carefully check your source to make certain that it is authentic. Legend says "receiving a bayberry candle as a gift and burning it down on New Year's Eve will insure many friends, good health, and excellent luck for the coming year."

Artificial Waxes

• Paraffin is made from mineral oil and there is argument among candlemakers as to whether or not it is a natural wax. The argument, that it is natural, is that it is an organic substance. Those on the opposing side say it is artificial and inferior because it is made from petrol that has been put through an elaborate refinery process.

Paraffin is inexpensive and readily available. It is harder and more brittle than natural waxes and is a good choice for molded candles. It has a lower oil content and thus a higher melting point. It is also translucent and a favored choice for over-dipping candles. However, paraffin is more likely to smoke and not burn as cleanly as the previously listed waxes. Some candlemakers have reported a nauseating side effect when melting paraffin. Some believe that the petroleum and carbon combustion ends up in the air we breathe and leaves a black soot on walls and surfaces.

• Gel wax is convenient to use because of its melt and pour capabilities as well as its visual appeal. It is made from mineral oil that is combined with substantial amounts of thermoplastic resin and butylated hydroxy toluene. Gel wax is not the most appropriate choice of wax for an aromatherapy candle and is somewhat incompatible with the idea of using natural essential oils in an artificial wax.

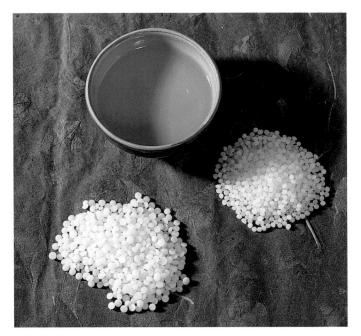

Wax additives

Wax Additives

A wide variety of wax additives are available, helping with a variety of candlemaking problems. They can increase luster, make wax more pliable, conserve the color, and aid in mold release. Most therapy-oriented candlemakers prefer to keep their candles as natural as possible and normally do fine without additives. However, if you are facing a particular problem in your candle creating, an additive might hold the answer.

• Luster crystals provide a brilliant sheen and opaqueness, as well as a longer-burning candle. The recommended use is 1 teaspoon per pound of wax.

• Microcrystallines are highly refined waxes and are used to change the properties of the carrier wax. A wide variety of microcrystallines are available and can be divided into two types. One type is pliable and is used to increase the elasticity of wax for modeling, as well as enhancing its ability to adhere. The other type makes the wax harder, increasing the durability of the candles. Adding more than 2% of the microcrystallines can cause wick and burning problems.

• Snow wax makes candle wax opaque with a high luster and prevents hot-weather sag. It also improves the surface texture and the burning time. Recommended use is 1 teaspoon per pound of wax. It is recommended that snow wax be melted separately, then mixed into melted candle wax.

• Snowflake oil is used for a decorative element and creates the beautiful snowflake effect common in many purchased aromatic candles. Follow the manufacturer's directions for the recommended amount.

• Stearic acid is added to paraffin to improve the candle's burning time as well as giving it a more opaque appearance. The recommended use is 2–5 tablespoons per pound of wax.

• Vybar makes candle wax harder, more opaque, and cuts down on the amount of shrinkage that takes place. It also serves as a fixative for the scent. Recommended use is no more than 2 teaspoons per pound. Begin with one teaspoon and do not exceed recommended amount.

Candle Molds

Candle molds come in an endless variety of shapes and sizes and are made of acrylic, metal, plastic, or rubber. Molds are relatively inexpensive and they can be used repeatedly.

Common household items such as cartons and containers will also make excellent molds. Anything from paper milk cartons to smooth-sided aluminum cans can be used as molds. Simply make a hole in the bottom center of cartons and containers with an awl or drill to thread the wick through. Secure wick as you would for a purchased mold, following the instructions for Making a Basic Molded Candle on page 26.

Make your own mold from a piece of corrugated cardboard.

1. Coat the corrugated side of the cardboard with vegetable oil.

2. Shape the cardboard into a round, square, or triangular mold as desired with corrugated side in.

3. Wrap shipping tape around the outside of the cardboard to hold its shape.

4. Make hole in lid.

5. Using mold sealer, secure bottom edge of cardboard to a plastic container lid.

6. Thread wick through hole in the plastic lid and secure.

7. Pour melted wax into mold.

8. When wax is set, tear away cardboard to reveal candle.

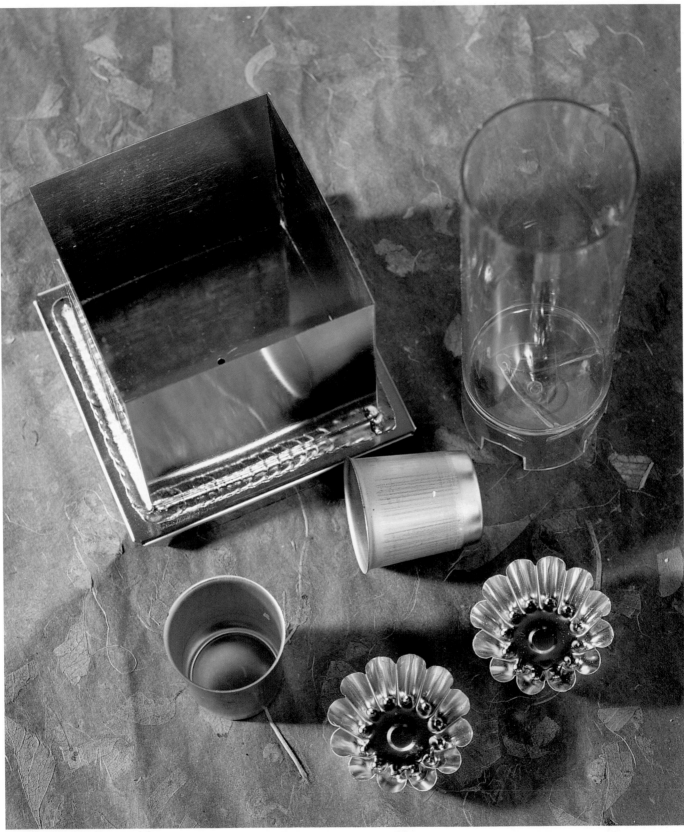

Various candle molds

Cleaning Molds

Candle molds should be clean and free from previous candle wax before using. Avoid scraping or scratching inside of molds when cleaning them, it will mar future candles. Glass, plastic, or metal candle molds may be cleaned in any one of the following ways:

• Fill sink with hot water and add liquid dish detergent. Allow candle molds to soak in water for 10 minutes. Wash candle molds, rinse, and dry thoroughly.

• Preheat oven to 200°F, and place paper toweling on a cookie sheet. Place the candle molds upside down on paper towels and place in oven for 7–8 minutes. Remove the cookie sheet from oven and wipe all excess wax from the inside of the candle molds.

• Clean metal molds with a candle mold cleaner, following the manufacturer's directions.

Candle Wicks

The wick must be carefully selected for the type of candle that you are making to insure proper burning. Wicks come in four basic types:

• Flat-braided wicks are best used in dipped taper candles. Note: Always use this wick with braid v's facing to the top of the candle. This prevents carbonized balls from forming on the end of the wick.

• Paper-core wicks are used for container candles, votives, and tea lights. However, they have a tendency to smoke more than other wicks.

• Square-braided wicks are sturdier than flat-braided wicks and are used in pillar candles.

• Wire-core wicks are primarily used for container candles, votives, and tea lights. Some wire-core wicks come pretabbed and need only to be anchored to the bottom of the mold or container. Caution: The metal core in these wicks is typically made from zinc, although you may find some with lead, and may contain hazardous fumes when burned.

Wicks that have been primed work best. Wicks can be purchased primed or unprimed. If the wicks are not primed, you can prime the wick by soaking it in melted wax for five minutes. Remove the wick from the wax and lay straight on waxed paper and allow to cool.

Size (or diameter) and length of the wick is usually determined by the diameter and length of the candle. Wick size is also determined by the type of wax that is used in the candle. Long-burning wax, such as beeswax or paraffin with hardening additives, will require a larger-sized wick.

The size of the wick is determined by the diameter of the finished candle, a small-sized wick for candles up to 2" in diameter, a medium-sized wick for 2"–3" candles, and a large-sized wick for 3"–4" candles. A smaller-sized wick may be used for votive candles.

The length of the wick is determined by measuring the height of the mold and adding 2". In some cases, you may wish to leave a longer wick that can be knotted or embellished with beads and charms for a more decorative effect or for gift giving.

Oftentimes, a poorly burning candle is caused by selecting the wrong wick for the diameter of the candle or the wax from which it is formed. To achieve consistent results, keep notes and document what works in the various candles you create.

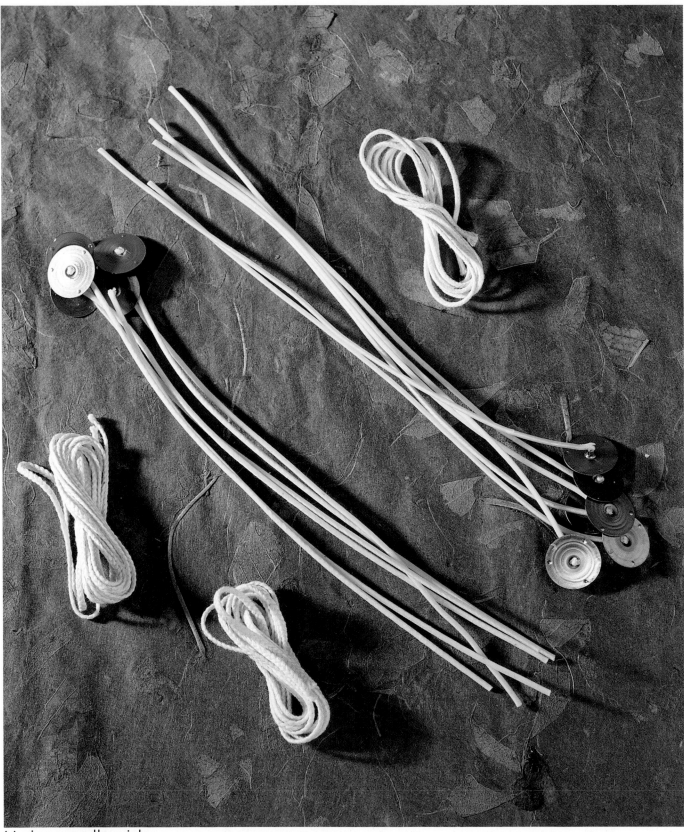

Various candle wicks

Candle Wick Tabs

Candle wick tabs are small metal disks to which the wicks may be attached for secure placement in a candle. A small amount of melted wax is poured into the bottom center of the mold. The disk is then centered in wax and secured as wax cools. Remainder of wax is then poured into the mold.

Candle Dyes

Candle dyes are available in liquid, solid, and powdered form. Add the dye a little at a time until desired color is achieved, following manufacturer's directions.

• Liquid dye is added to the melted wax and blends in quite easily.

• Solid dye consists of concentrated color pigment and wax. The tablets (or chips) should be cut up, then added to the melted wax and stirred until fully melted.

• Powdered candle pigments should be dissolved in warmed stearic acid before being mixed into melted wax. Powdered pigments are so concentrated that only a very small amount is required for coloring wax.

Adding Essential Oils

The information addressed at the beginning of this chapter covers many of the details concerning the use and benefits of essential oils. There are a few other details that need to be kept in mind when using essential oils:

• Citrus oils may cause a flare-up in burning candles, with orange being the worst. When using these oils, they should be included in quantities of less than 5%. It is a good idea to test the citrus oils in sample candles.

• Essential oils made from spices are as intense and powerful as the spices themselves and should always be used sparingly. They may cause the flame to sputter as well as overwhelm the sense of smell. Never use ground spice in the core of the candle because it may congest the wick.

• Several of the pricier essential oils, such as jasmine, rose, and sandalwood, are often sold in dilution or as a synthetically manufactured fragrance. Always purchase oils from a trusted source. Because of their expense, these oils are best used in small amounts in a candle or in an aroma lamp or diffuser.

Using Purchased Candles

For projects calling for a pillar candle, a purchased candle may be substituted. Aromatic pillar candles are readily available in the marketplace and could be purchased in a scent compatible to those in the Essential Blend recommended for that project as a shortcut.

An unscented candle could also be purchased and scented with essential oils, using one of the following methods:

• Light candle and allow a pool of wax to form. Blow out the flame and add the Essential Blend to the pool of wax. As the wax cools, the essential oils are absorbed into the candle.

• Heat the end of an ice pick and make 3–4 holes around the wick in the candle core. Place drops of Essential Blend into holes and allow them to be absorbed into the wax for 20 minutes or more before lighting.

• This method works well for scenting tapers. Trim the wick to ¼". Place essential blend around the base of the wick and allow the oils to be absorbed into the wick for 20 minutes or more before lighting.

Wax Temperatures for Candlemaking

Acrylic molds	180°F–210°F
Bayberry candles	130°F
Container candles	160°F–165°F
Dipping candles	155°F–160°F
Glass molds	170°F–200°F
Metal molds	180°F–210°F
Rubber molds	160°F–180°F
Taper candles	158°F
Tear-away molds*	160°F

*(Such as corrugated cardboard)

Making a Basic Molded Candle

1. Clear work space and cover surface with waxed paper to protect against drips or spills. Caution: Avoid wax drips or spills on burners or range at all costs because of the flammability of the wax. Never pour wax into a pan sitting on burner.

2. Determine amount of mold blend wax needed to fill mold by filling mold with water and measuring the water. 3 ounces of wax is equivalent to 3 ½ ounces of water.

3. Place wax into large garbage bag and onto a solid surface. Using hammer and screwdriver, break wax into small chunks.

4. Place wax chunks in top pan of double boiler.

5. Place double boiler on range and heat water in bottom pan to boiling point. As wax begins to melt and pool, place thermometer into wax but do not allow it to touch bottom of pan.

6. Reduce heat to medium low so that water continues at a gentle boil. Note: Do not allow water to boil dry.

7. While wax is melting, prepare mold by lightly coating inside of mold with mold release.

8. Cut wick to desired length. See Candle Wicks on pages 23–24 to determine type, size, and length of wick.

9. Thread wick through hole in bottom of mold. Cover hole and secure end of wick to outside of mold with mold sealer to prevent leakage.

10. Pull wick straight up through mold, placing metal skewer on top of mold. Make certain that wick is centered and taut, then wrap wick around metal skewer.

11. When wax is melted to proper temperature, add desired additives to the melted wax. See Wax Temperatures for Candlemaking at left. See Wax Additives on pages 20–21.

12. Add candle dye and stir until color is evenly distributed.

13. Add essential blend to wax when ready to pour. If wax is too hot, some of the oil may dissipate and some scent may be lost.

avoid making a line around outside edge of the candle. Allow wax to cool.

16. Remove skewer and mold sealer from ends of mold. Tip mold upside down and candle should slide out on its own. Note: If candle does not slide out on its own, place mold in freezer for 5–10 minutes. Remove mold from freezer and slide candle out.

17. Trim bottom end of wick flush with candle. Trim top of wick to ½". Note: Wick may be left longer for a decorative effect.

Over-dipping Candles

Over-dipping candles is done in a dipping can, a tall cylindrical metal container that can be purchased in a craft or candlemaking store.

1. Melt wax to 165°F and color. See Making a Basic Molded Candle on page 26. Note: The color for over-dipping must be intense and may need at the very least, double the amount of dye necessary for a regular candle.

2. Pour melted wax into the dipping can and, holding candle by the wick, dip candle once into and out of wax. Allow to cool.

3. Dip candle two more times, allowing it to cool between dippings.

Chunk Candle

Creating chunks for the chunk candle is done by simply cutting wax into pieces from

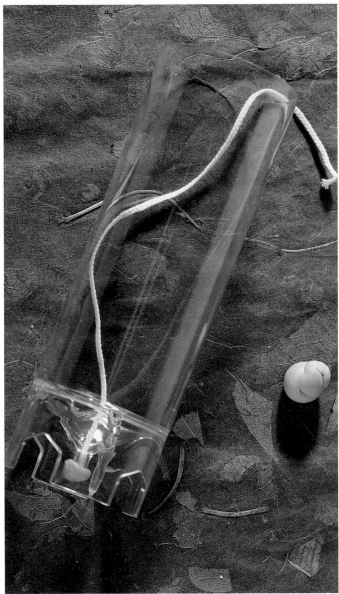
Mold with mold sealer and wick.

14. Slowly pour melted wax into mold until mold is 90% full. Pour excess wax into a small can and set aside. Lightly tap mold to release any air bubbles. Allow wax to cool. Note: As wax cools, an indentation may form around the wick.

15. Place small can of wax into water of bottom pan of double boiler and remelt wax. Fill indentation with melted wax. Note: Fill only to top of indentation to

wax that has been scented and dyed. The wax should be molded in a shallow container to cut more easily.

1. Melt wax to 194°–198° F and color, See Making a Basic Molded Candle on pages 26–27.

2. Pour wax to a depth of ½"–1" into shallow plastic container.

3. Allow wax to set and remove from container. Using sharp kitchen knife, cut wax chunks into 1" pieces or as desired.

Candle Tips

• Candles should always be left to cure at least 24 hours before being lit.

• Always melt wax in a double boiler or water bath. Never melt wax and leave it unattended over direct heat. Wax will self-ignite when overheated.

• Do not extinguish burning wax with water. Instead, smother the flames with baking soda, a towel, a lid, or a blanket.

• Always clean up spills as they happen. Melted wax, collecting in the proximity of a burner, is a fire hazard.

• Never pour wax down a drain because it will clog the drain.

• If hot wax is spilled on skin, do not wipe it off. Rinse the skin under cold water and allow the wax to set up and then scrape it off.

• Remove uncolored wax from fabric by allowing it to harden and then scraping it off; or place a paper napkin or facial tissue over and under the wax spot. Iron it with a hot iron. If the wax is dyed, it would be better to have it professionally dry-cleaned so the color is not set into the fabric by the heat of the iron. There are new products on the market that could aid in the removal of wax from fabric and other surfaces.

• Use pots and containers that are dedicated to candlemaking. Retire these items from food use. Consider purchasing pots and containers from thrift stores or at garage sales.

• Waxy residues can be removed by placing the container in the fridge or freezer until the wax becomes loose and is easily removed. See Cleaning Molds on page 23.

• Save all candle leftovers because they are valuable raw materials and be can remelted and used again. Let your friends know that you collect leftover candle odds and ends.

• Always be aware of flowers, ribbons, and other decorative items that are in close proximity of a candle flame. Never leave a candle unattended.

Troubleshooting

Candle burning straight down the middle

• A candle made from a hard wax will burn straight down the wick, leaving the sides of the candle unmelted. The cavity created will make it difficult for the flame to sustain itself. A softer wax, such as a container wax, could be used. However, using a wax with a lower melting point may create a pool of melted wax around the base of a pillar candle.

- A small, similarly scented votive or tea light could be placed in the cavity.

Candle color changes

- Wax was too hot when color was added. Avoid heating wax that will be colored above 190°F.

- Candle was exposed to direct sunlight. Many colors fade in sunlight. UV-protective additives are available.

Candle stops burning

- Additives such as colors, spices, or essential oils of inferior quality can clog the wick.

Candle will not burn

- The wick was not primed. Saturate the wick with liquid wax or light it upside down to allow melted wax to prime wick.

Candle will not release from mold

- Make certain to coat the mold with a mold release.

- A high percentage of beeswax may produce a candle that is sticky or does not shrink enough for easy release. Beeswax is less than ideal for using in molded candles.

- Place mold into freezer or refrigerator for 5–10 minutes. Remove and check to see if candle releases.

- The candle may be run under hot water for release, although this may cause imperfections on the candle surface.

- Add extra stearic acid into melted wax to aid in mold release.

- Check molds for pits or dents.

Container candles leaving excess wax on container walls

- Container candles burn best when they are lit for a minimum of four hours at a time. Burning a candle for short periods of time will cause unburned wax on container walls.

- Use a container wax or a wax with a lower burning point.

- Use a larger wick size.

Cracked surface

- Candle was cooled too fast.

- Candle was left in freezer too long.

Dripping candle

- Wick is too small, it may not be able to absorb the amount of wax melting around it.

- Wick is the wrong type for the wax blend.

- Wick is not properly centered. Check the position of the wick after candle is out and manually center it, if possible.

- The wax used was too soft and had too low of a melting point.

- Check for a draft around the flame.

Outside of candle looks old or dusty

• Polish the outside of the candle with a nylon stocking or almond oil.

• Over-dip candle to renew its look.

Pits and bubbles

• Wax may have been too cold when poured.

• Wax was poured too fast.

• Mold release was applied too heavily in the mold.

• Too much essential blend was added.

• Mold should be clean and dust-free before pouring wax.

Scent in candle is not strong enough

• Wax was too hot when scent was added.

• Allow candle to burn one hour before judging strength of scent, because scent primarily rises from the liquid wax pool.

• Rubbing hands over the outside of a candle should activate scent in a candle that lost fragrance in the outer layer.

• Add extra essential blend to candle. See Using Purchased Candles on pages 25–26.

• Be certain to add Essential Blend to melted wax at the last minute before pouring the candle into a mold or container.

• Increase the amount of Essential Blend the next time the candle is created.

• Add up to 1% Vybar to the melted wax the next time the candle is created. Vybar serves as a fixative, but too much Vybar will bind the molecules and not allow any scent to be released. Note: Some "one-pour" waxes already contain Vybar.

Shrink Wells

• This is a normal occurrence in paraffin wax blends. The wax shrinks as it cools and an indentation is formed around the wick. Make certain to retain excess wax, then remelt and pour wax into indentation. Repeat if necessary.

• Occasionally, the shrink well comes at the bottom of the candle. You can straighten the bottom of the candle by trimming it off or melting it flat on a foiled-covered frying pan.

• Beeswax can be added to paraffin in a 1:4 ratio to eliminate shrinkage; however, this will require a larger size wick than paraffin candles of the same size.

• Use a "one-pour" paraffin wax compound or an additive, such as Vybar, which reduces the amount of shrinkage, but may have some affect on candle performance.

Sides of candle cave in

• Air bubbles may be trapped inside candle. This problem can be prevented by tapping mold or poking a skewer around the wick to eliminate bubbles immediately after pouring candle.

Smoking candle

- Wick is too thick.

- Wick is the wrong type for the wax blend.

- Wick may be too long. Trim wick to ¼".

- Check for drafts around the flame.

Sputtering flame

- Wick is drawing from an air or oil pocket that has formed in the candle. This problem can be prevented by tapping mold or poking a skewer around the wick to eliminate bubbles immediately after pouring candle.

- Pouring with a container that is wet on the outside may allow water to drop inside wax and form a water pocket.

- Too much spicy essential oil added.

Unintentional mottling or snowflake pattern

- Wax too cold when poured.

- Candle cooled too slowly.

- Too much palm wax or stearic acid.

- Too much Essential Blend was added.

- Add up to 1% Vybar to reduce or eliminate the effect.

Wax buildup and dirty molds

- Clean molds, following suggestions in Cleaning Molds on page 23.

Weak flame or drowning wick

- Wick is too small.

- Wick is too loose in the candle.

- Melting point of the wax is too high for the size of wick used.

- Add less stearic acid or other additives the next time the candle is created.

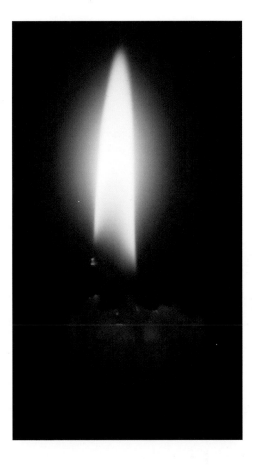

LIGHTEN UP

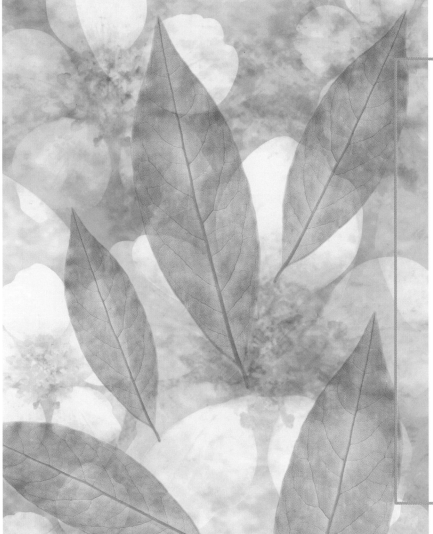

To create a specific environment, to enhance your state of body and mind, to incorporate the five elements of feng shui—you must tend to all of the five senses not just the sense of smell.

To lighten up in addition to your soothing blends of lavender or vanilla for relaxing, surround yourself with the calming color of blue, eat comfort food, sit in a chair covered with a plush or velvet throw, and listen to quiet or very soft music. It is important that all of the senses help in achieving that state of body and mind that you desire.

Ban stress and anxiety from your life. . . . Relaxation holds the key to well being in the 21st century. We all have an overabundance of demands and worries in our life so for the sake of our health it is important to be soothed by the nourishments of nature. The simple aroma of a tangy bergamot, the sun-drenched essence of French lavender, or the sweet flavor of the precious orchid fruit vanilla can return you to a state of harmony. Aromatherapy is: following your nose into a mini vacation—a superb moment of joy and peace.

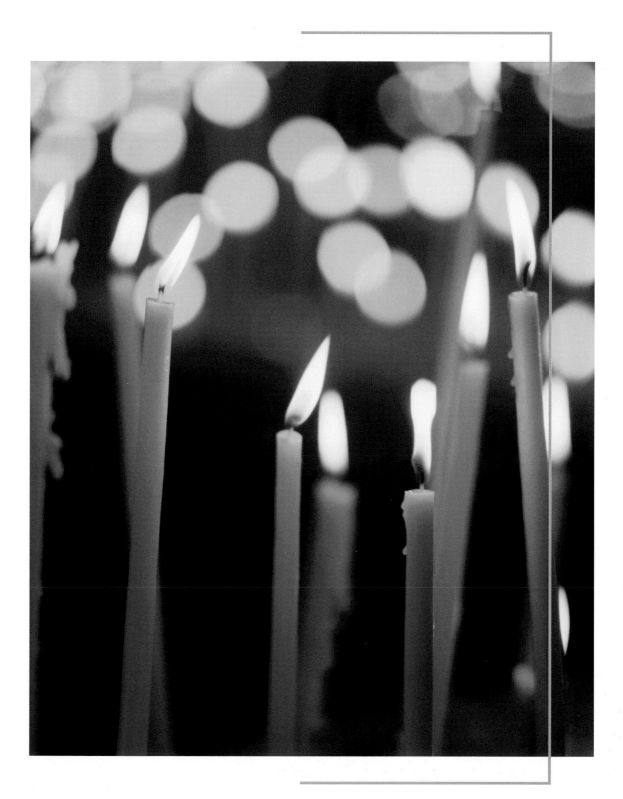

SMOOTH VANILLA

double boiler
essential oils: sandalwood, vanilla
kitchen scale
metal pouring pot
metal skewer
mold: round pillar
mold release
mold sealer
mold-blend wax
primed wick: square-braided
scissors
small tin container
thermometer

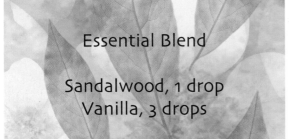

Essential Blend

Sandalwood, 1 drop
Vanilla, 3 drops

VANILLA has a base note with a very mild and soothing scent. The smooth vanilla scent is one that is spiritually warming and calming. Derived from an orchid seedpod, and used in tincture form to flavor, vanilla offers a rich, grounding fragrance to any blend. It relaxes the mind and body and diffuses irritability and angst.

pillar candle

1 Using double boiler, melt wax.

2 Using mold release, lightly coat inside of candle mold.

3 Cut wick to appropriate length and thread through hole in bottom of mold and secure.

4 Pour melted wax into metal pouring pot.

5 Add essential blend to melted wax.

6 Pour melted wax into mold until 90% full. Pour excess wax into tin container. Allow wax to set.

7 Remelt excess wax and fill indentation. Allow wax to set.

8 Tip mold upside down and remove candle.

9 Trim wick at top and bottom of candle.

Vanilla blends well with:
    clove
    sandalwood
    vetiver

Other benefits and uses for vanilla:
    calms nerves
    reduces muscle tension
    revitalizes the body

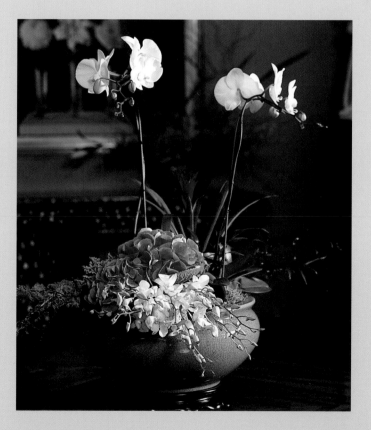

embedded marble candle

1 Using double boiler, melt wax.

2 Using mold release, lightly coat inside of candle mold.

3 Scent white pillar candle with essential blend. See Using Purchased Candles, pages 25–26.

4 Center pillar candle in mold.

5 Drop glass marbles into mold until half the height of candle is full.

6 Pour melted wax into metal pouring pot.

7 Add essential blend to melted wax.

8 Slowly pour melted wax over marbles until 90% full. Pour excess wax into tin container. Allow wax to set.

9 Remelt excess wax and fill mold with melted wax. Allow wax to set. Note: Do not pour melted wax above top edge of pillar candle.

10 Tip mold upside down and remove candle.

tip

Using a heat gun, some wax may be melted away to partially expose some glass marbles, giving a decorative uneven finish.

Lavender blends well with:
- chamomile
- citrus
- lemongrass
- rose

Other benefits and uses for lavender:
- disinfects
- enhances sleep
- loosens congestion
- reduces muscle tension
- reduces pain
- repels insects
- soothes and heals skin

LAVENDER

has a middle note with a floral scent. The floral scent is one that is clean and fresh, as well as being one of the most versatile essential oils. Lavender has been used for centuries for scenting linens and bathing. It can be used topically as well as a scent, and washes away physical and mental impurities. The flower is as multifaceted as the extracted oil. The flower buds can be used to make a tea for headaches and nervous exhaustion, or as filler for a scented pillow. The oil is uplifting, soothing, balancing, and an antidepressant. It can dispel irritability and melancholy, relieves stress, and is good for shock, heart palpitations, dizziness, and some PMS symptoms.

Essential Blend

Clary sage, 1 drop
Lavender, 2 drops
Lemon, 2 drops

LIFTING LAVENDER

double boiler
essential oils: clary sage, lavender, lemon
glass marbles or pebbles
kitchen scale
metal pouring pot
metal spoon
mold: round pillar (larger then unscented pillar candle)
mold release
mold-blend wax
small tin container
thermometer
unscented pillar candle, white (in the photograph at the right, the inner candle was approximately 3" x 6")

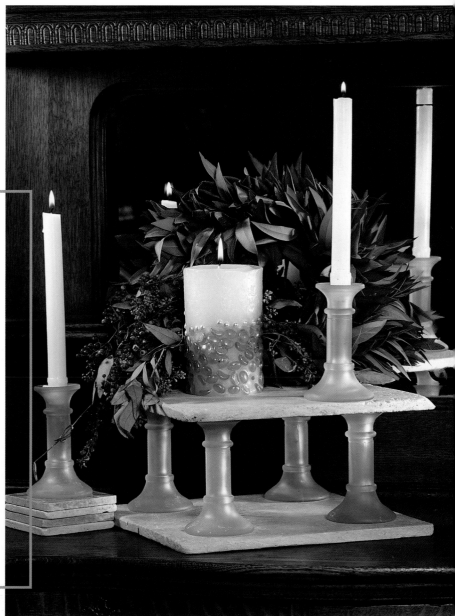

string-wrapped pillar

1 Using double boiler, melt wax.

2 Using mold release, lightly coat inside of candle mold.

3 Cut wick to appropriate length and thread through hole in bottom of mold and secure.

4 Pour melted wax into metal pouring pot.

5 Add orange dye to melted wax.

6 Add essential blend to melted wax.

7 Pour melted wax into mold until 90% full. Pour excess wax into tin container. Allow wax to set.

8 Remelt excess wax and fill indentation. Allow wax to set.

9 Tip mold upside down and remove candle.

10 Wrap candle with string, starting at bottom of candle and wrapping in a spiraling motion toward top. Secure ends with small amount of melted wax.

11 Press seashells into sides of candle at top, using melted wax to secure.

12 Pour melted wax into dipping vat. Holding candle by wick at top, dip into wax. Hold for a few seconds and lift out and allow to set.

13 Trim wick at top and bottom of candle.

Orange blends well with:
- cinnamon
- cypress
- juniper
- sandalwood

Other benefits and uses for orange:
- antidepressant
- purifies body and mind
- reduces muscle tension
- relieves anxiety and fear

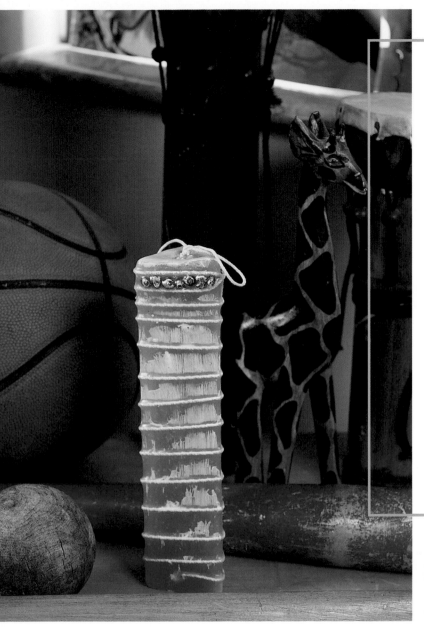

CITRUS HIGH

double boiler
dye: orange
essential oils: cedarwood, orange,
    ylang-ylang
kitchen scale
metal pouring pot
metal skewer
metal spoon
mold: tall triangular
    pillar
mold release
mold sealer
mold-blend wax
primed wick: square-braided
scissors
seashells
small tin container
string
tall dipping vat
thermometer

Essential Blend

Cedarwood, 5 drops
Orange, 3 drops
Ylang-ylang, 1 drop

ORANGE has a top note with a fresh citrus scent. This scent relaxes, balances, and heals. Orange is used to uplift and energize the mind and spirit; it can help to ease feelings of depression and hopelessness. It is a cheerful scent that will have a powerful effect on the spirit's well being.

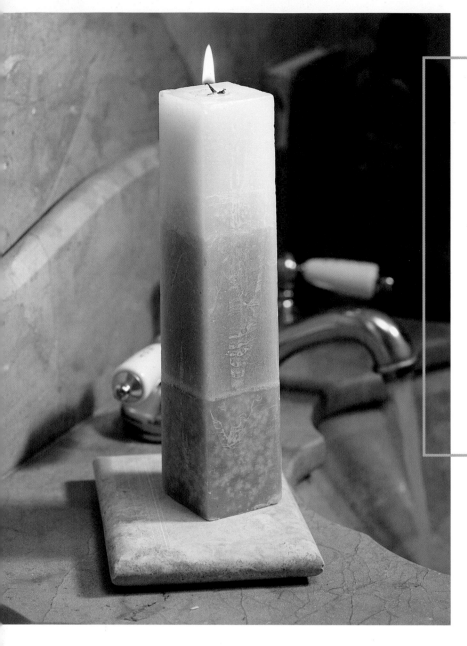

SUMMERY SAGE

double boiler
dyes: brown, green, ivory
essential oils: cedarwood, clary sage,
    grapefruit
kitchen scale
metal pouring pot
metal skewer
mold: triangle pillar
mold release
mold sealer
mold-blend wax
primed wick: square-braided
small metal containers (3)
small tin container
thermometer

Essential Blend

Cedarwood, 3 drops
Clary sage, 3 drops
Grapefruit, 6 drops

CLARY SAGE has a top to middle note with a fresh, sweet scent. This scent is one that calms, eases pain, and reduces tension and stress. It warms and stimulates the body, and promotes restful sleep. Clary sage has also been noted for its uplifting and regenerating effect on the mind and body. This harmonious and herbaceous oil will encourage joy and relaxation, bringing a sense of peaceful bliss and balance to those who experience it.

layered pillar

1 Using double boiler, melt wax.

2 Using mold release, lightly coat inside of candle mold.

3 Cut wick to appropriate length and thread through hole in bottom of mold and secure.

4 Pour ⅓ of melted wax into metal pouring pot.

5 Add green dye to melted wax in metal pouring pot.

6 Divide essential blend into 3 parts and add one part to melted wax in metal pouring pot.

7 Pour melted wax into mold until ⅓ full. Allow wax to set.

8 Pour ½ of remaining melted wax into metal pouring pot and add brown dye.

9 Add one part of essential blend to melted wax as in Step 6.

10 Pour melted wax into mold until ⅔ full. Allow wax to set.

11 Pour remaining melted wax into metal pouring pot and add ivory dye.

12 Add remaining part of essential blend to melted wax.

13 Pour melted wax into mold until completely full. Allow wax to set.

14 Remelt excess ivory wax and fill indentation. Allow wax to set.

15 Tip mold upside down and remove candle.

16 Trim wick at top and bottom of candle.

Clary sage blends well with:
  geranium
  jasmine
  lavender
  orange

Other benefits and uses for clary sage:
  antidepressant
  relieves stress

CITRONELLA DELIGHT

bay leaves
dipping vat
double boiler
dye: brown
essential oils: citronella, lavender,
    lemongrass
glue pen with sponge applicator
kitchen scale
sage-green ribbon
taper-blend wax
thermometer
unscented pillar candle, ivory (3" x 6")
urn planter
waxed paper

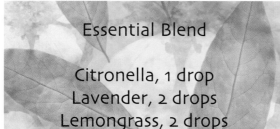

Essential Blend

Citronella, 1 drop
Lavender, 2 drops
Lemongrass, 2 drops

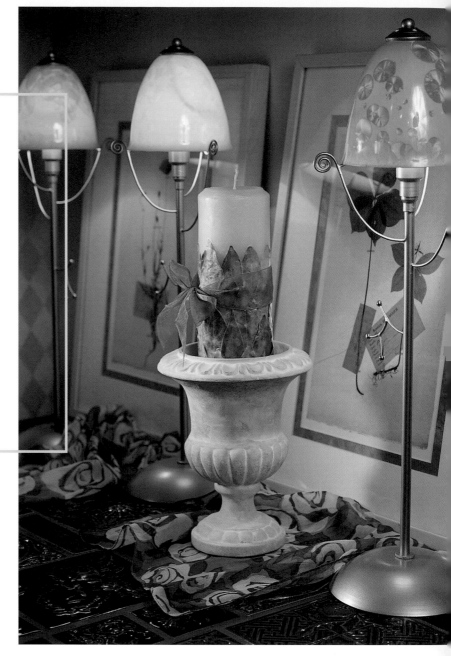

CITRONELLA
has a middle to top note with a sweet citrusy scent. Citronella is known for its powerful insect repelling qualities and is favored for use in outdoor garden candles. Citronella's fresh and fruity properties will help ease headache, and help eliminate fatigue.

dipped bayleaf candle

1

Apply glue to backs of bay leaves. Adhere leaves to pillar candle. Note: Leaves can be carefully repositioned if glue is still wet. Allow glue to dry.

2

Using double boiler, melt wax.

3

Scent pillar candle with essential blend. See Using Purchased Candles on pages 25–26. Note: A round pillar candle could be made and scented with essential blend.

4

Pour melted wax into dipping vat.

5

Add dye to melted wax.

6

Holding candle by wick, dip candle into dipping vat in one smooth motion. Repeat dipping two additional times. Place on waxed paper and allow to set.

7

Tie ribbon around candle and set in urn.

tip

Dipping wax may also be scented with essential blend.

Citronella blends well with:
    clove
    jasmine
    juniper berry
    nutmeg
    vetiver

Other benefits and uses for citronella:
    soothes body and mind
    uplifting

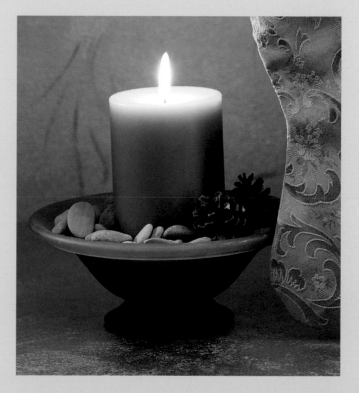

candle melts

1 Using double boiler, melt wax.

2 Using mold release, lightly coat inside of candle mold.

3 Pour melted wax into pouring pot.

4 Add dye to melted wax.

5 Add essential blend to melted wax.

6 Place dried lavender into melted wax and stir.

7 Pour melted wax into mold until full. Allow wax to set up.

8 Tip mold upside down and remove candle.

Ginger blends well with:
    lavender
    lemon
    lime
    neroli
    orange
    rosewood

Other benefits and uses for ginger:
    enhances appetite
    heightens senses
    relieves stress
    soothes body and mind

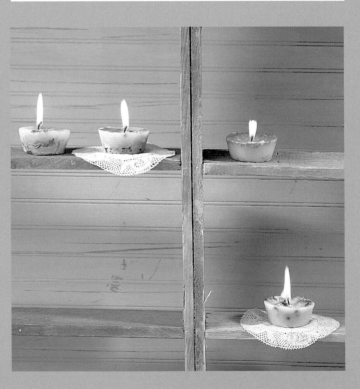

GINGER

has a middle to top note with an earthy and spicy aroma. It is lightening to the senses and warming to the soul. Ginger is believed to be high in yang energy by the Chinese. This spicy root is used for flavoring foods as well as for medicinal purposes.

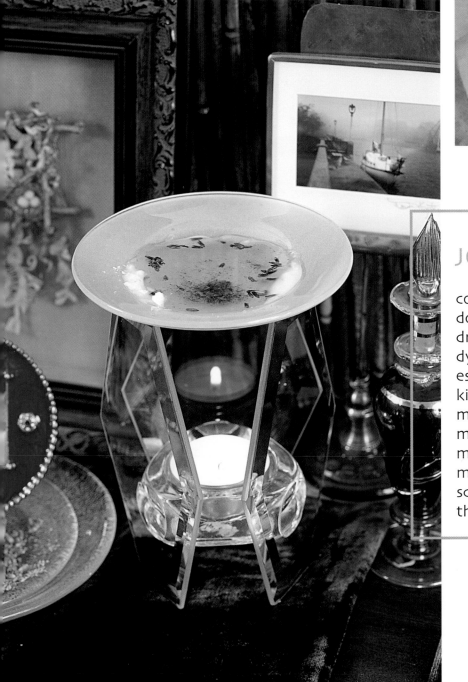

Essential Blend

Ginger, 2 drops
Lavender, 2 drops
Neroli, 1 drop

JOLLY GINGER

container-blend wax
double boiler
dried lavender
dye: white
essential oils: ginger, lavender, neroli
kitchen scale
metal pouring pot
metal spoon
mold: tea light
mold release
scissors
thermometer

AWAKEN YOUR SENSES

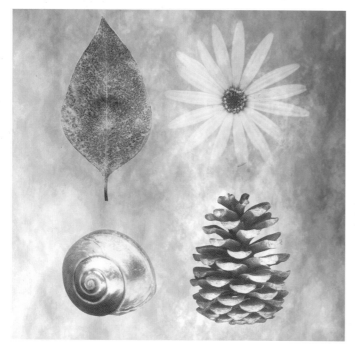

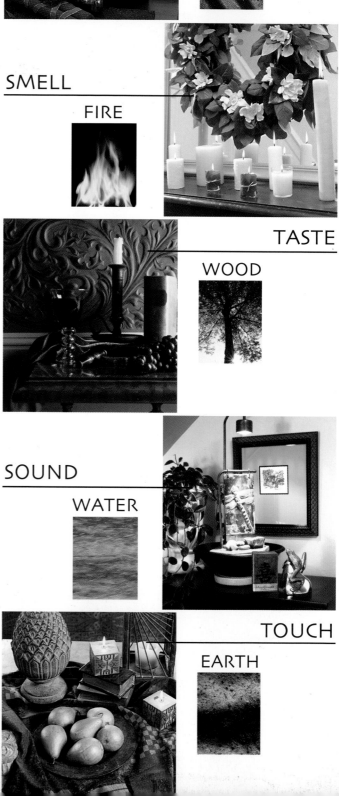

SIGHT
METAL

SMELL
FIRE

TASTE
WOOD

SOUND
WATER

TOUCH
EARTH

The five elements of feng shui—metal, fire, wood, water, and earth—are elements of energy which balance your environment and promote certain qualities. Each relates to a certain power and a particular season: water has the powers of release and renewal and relates to winter; wood is personal growth and relates to spring; fire is the power of expansion and transformation and relates to summer; earth is grounding and a support energy and relates to early autumn; and metal is the energy of the mind and relates to late summer. Depending on your own individual needs these qualities can help you create certain environments, establish different moods, and develop certain types of activities.

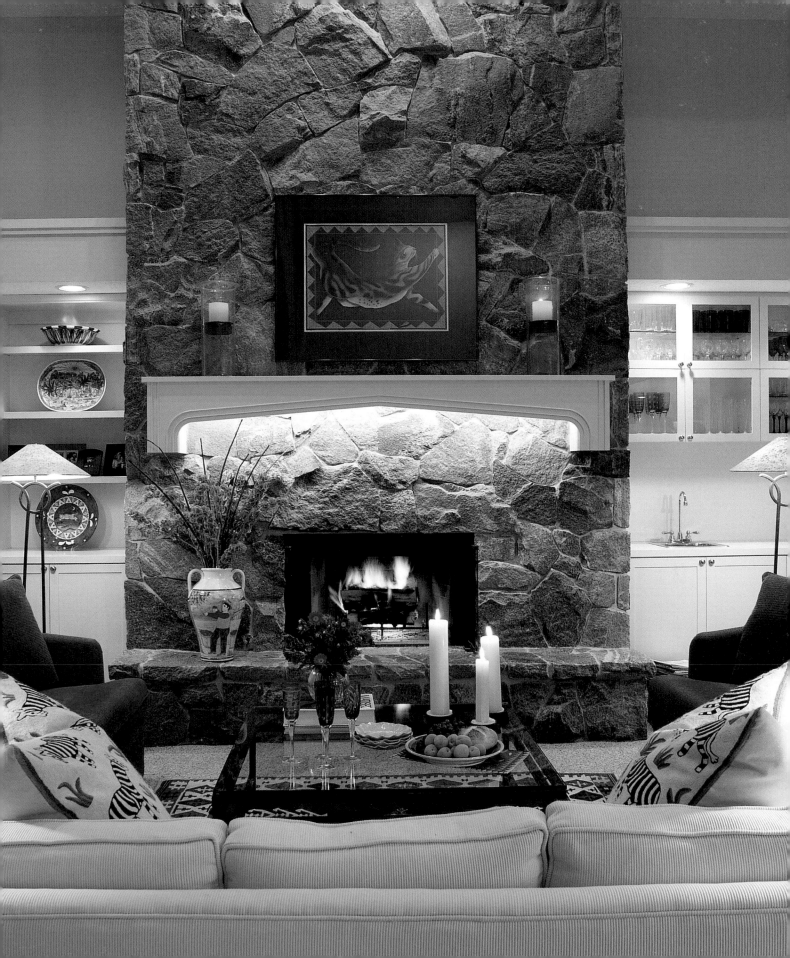

FIRE UP

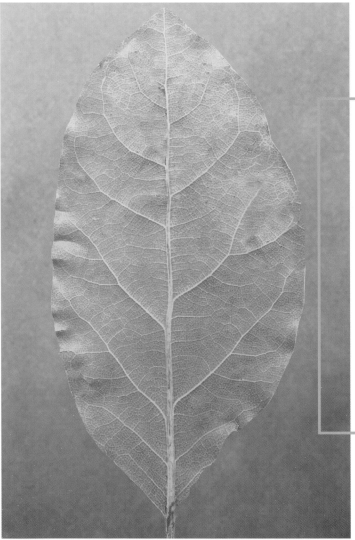

Increase your energy and your concentration by tending to all of the senses. Surround yourself with uplifting music, sit in a room that is painted a vibrant warm color, eat natural fruits that are high in sugar, sit in a chair that is covered in vibrant tactile fabrics, and surround yourself with the essential blends of aromatherapy.

Enjoy abundant energy and concentration. . . . Whether you are worn out by long hours of work or need help getting into gear after sleeping or eating, turn to essential oils for a pick-me-up and a little boost of energy. The oils recommended in this chapter are strong stimulants and will leave you rejuvenated and energized.

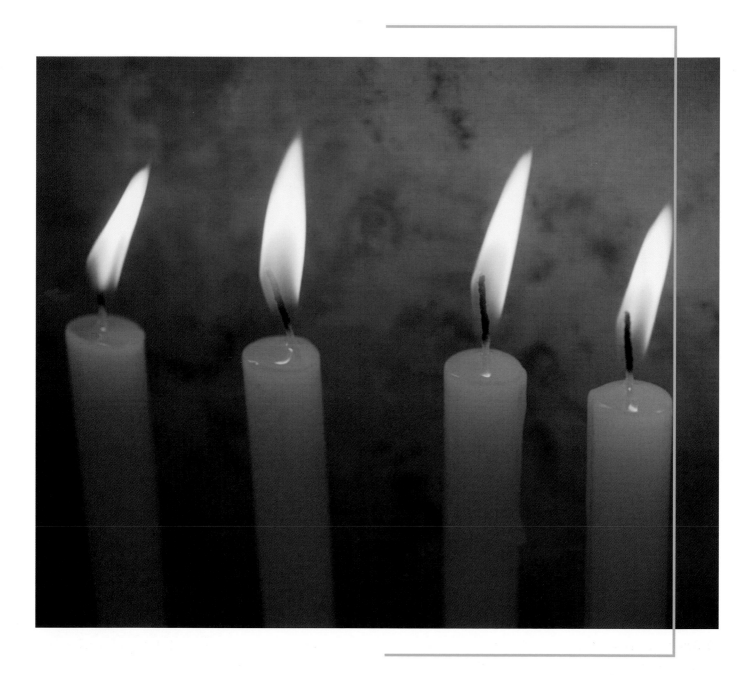

rustic candle

1 Using double boiler, melt wax.

2 Using mold release, lightly coat inside of candle mold.

3 Cut wick to appropriate length and thread through hole in bottom of mold and secure.

4 Pour melted wax into metal pouring pot.

5 Add ivory dye to melted wax.

6 Add essential blend to melted wax.

7 Pour melted wax into mold until 90% full. Pour excess wax into tin container. Allow wax to set.

8 Remelt excess wax and fill indentation. Allow wax to set.

9 Tip mold upside down and remove candle.

10 Trim wick at top and bottom of candle.

11 Using palette knife, daub acrylic texture medium onto candle to create a textured look, following manufacturer's directions. Allow to dry.

12 Paint with liquid iron, carefully filling in between spaces in texture medium. Allow to dry.

13 Apply rusting compound to textured area of candle, following manufacturer's directions. Allow to rust and dry.

Cypress blends well with:
- juniper
- lavender
- lemon
- pine

Other benefits and uses for cypress:
- reduces muscle tension
- relieves stress
- stimulates circulation

FRESH CYPRESS

acrylic texture medium
disposable foam cup: large
double boiler
dye: ivory
essential oils: bergamot, cypress,
    petitgrain
ground liquid iron
kitchen scale
metal pouring pot
metal skewer
mold: cylindrical pillar
mold release
mold sealer
mold-blend wax
paintbrush (1")
palette knife
primed wick: square-braided
rusting compound
scissors
small tin container
thermometer

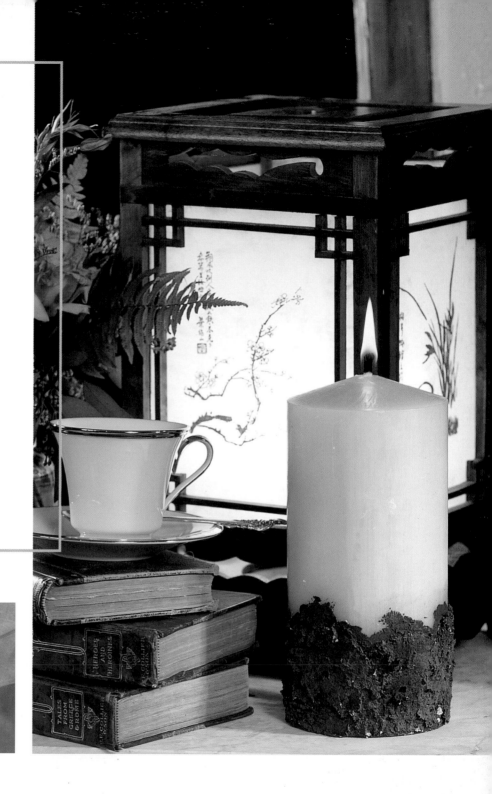

Essential Blend

Bergamot, 4 drops
Cypress, 5 drops
Petitgrain, 2 drops

CYPRESS has a middle note with a fresh woodsy scent. The cypress scent is one that promotes mental concentration. It is also spiritually calming and refreshing. Cypress helps to regulate female hormones and has also been known to reduce the appearance of cellulite. This warming and purifying aroma has the ability to rejuvenate and awaken the senses, to improve coping skills, relieve tension, and encourage restful sleep.

chunk candle

1 Using double boiler, melt wax.

2 Using mold release, lightly coat inside of candle mold.

3 Cut wick to appropriate length and thread through hole in bottom of mold and secure.

4 Position green wax chunks in candle mold as desired.

5 Pour melted wax into metal pouring pot.

6 Add essential blend to melted wax.

7 Pour melted wax into mold until 90% full. Pour excess wax into tin container. Allow wax to set.

8 Remelt excess wax and fill indentation. Allow wax to set.

9 Tip mold upside down and remove candle.

10 Trim wick at top and bottom of candle.

Peppermint blends well with:
  clove
  eucalyptus
  lime
  marjoram

Other benefits and uses for peppermint:
  improves digestion
  loosens congestion
  reduces fatigue
  reduces inflammation
  repels insects
  stimulates nerves

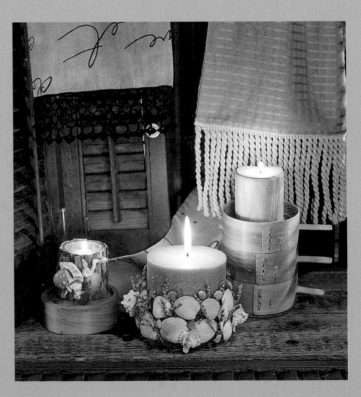

PEPPERMINT

has a top note with a very fresh and minty scent. This scent is one that stimulates and energizes the mind and body. It awakens the senses and encourages mental clarity. It has been noted to relieve pain and alleviate cold and flu symptoms such as dizziness, fever, headaches, and vomiting. Peppermint's refreshing qualities will uplift and enlighten the mood, and increase strength.

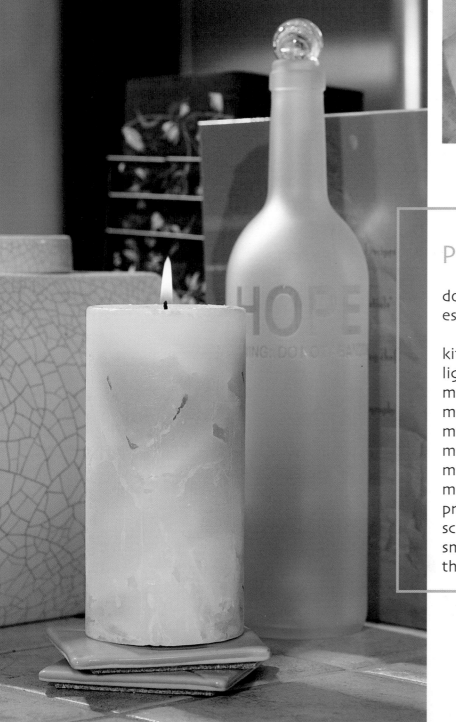

Essential Blend

Lavender, 2 drops
Peppermint, 4 drops
Rosemary, 3 drops

PEPPERMINT PATTY

double boiler
essential oils: lavender, peppermint, rosemary
kitchen scale
light green wax chunks
metal pouring pot
metal skewer
mold: round pillar
mold release
mold sealer
mold-blend wax
primed wick: square-braided
scissors
small tin container
thermometer

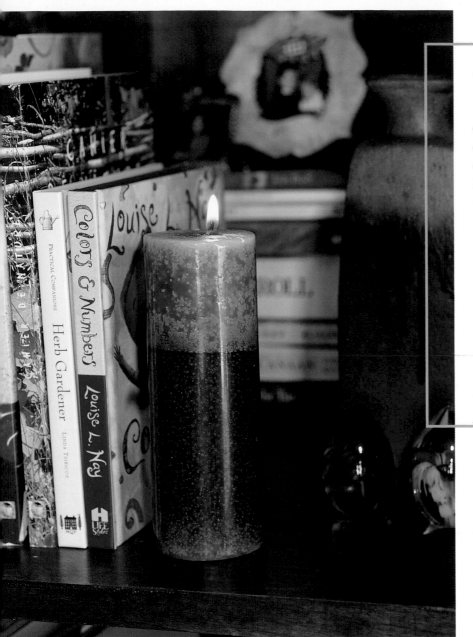

WOODY JUNIPER

double boiler
dyes: green, purple
essential oil: juniper berry
kitchen scale
metal pouring pot
metal skewer
mold: round pillar
mold release
mold sealer
mold-blend wax
primed wick: square-braided
scissors
small metal containers (2)
small tin container
thermometer

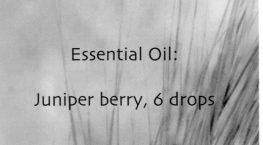

Essential Oil:

Juniper berry, 6 drops

JUNIPER BERRY has a middle note that is energizing and balancing. It improves concentration and mental clarity. Combined with elements of feng shui, juniper berry makes an ideal candle for intuition and self-cultivation. The color green signifies wood. Wood promotes growth, new beginnings, freshness, and nurturing. The color purple signifies prosperity.

feng shui layered candle

1 Using double boiler, melt wax.

2 Using mold release, lightly coat inside of candle mold.

3 Cut wick to appropriate length and thread through hole in bottom of mold and secure.

4 Pour ⅔ of melted wax into metal pouring pot.

5 Add purple dye to melted wax in metal pouring pot.

6 Divide essential oil into three parts and add two parts to melted wax in metal pouring pot.

7 Pour melted wax into mold until ⅓ full. Allow wax to set.

8 Pour remaining melted wax into metal pouring pot and add green dye.

9 Add remaining part of essential oil to melted wax as in Step 6.

10 Pour melted wax into mold until full. Allow wax to set.

11 Remelt any excess green wax and fill indentation with melted wax. Allow wax to set.

12 Tip mold upside down and remove candle.

13 Trim wick at top and bottom of candle.

Juniper berry blends well with:
    bergamot
    rosemary
    sandalwood

Other benefits and uses for juniper berry:
    purifies body and mind
    repels insects

dipped pinecones

1 Using double boiler, melt wax.

2 Pour melted wax into dipping pot.

3 Add dye to melted wax.

4 Add essential blend to melted wax.

5 Using slotted spoon, dip pinecone into wax and remove.

6 Place pinecone onto waxed paper. Allow to set.

7 Repeat for remaining pinecones.

tip
Use pinecones to light fireplace and add aroma to a room.

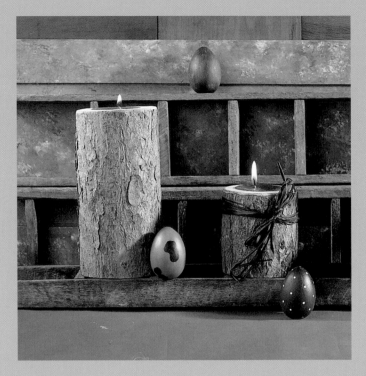

Spruce blends well with:
- lemon
- peppermint
- spearmint

Other benefits and uses for spruce:
- enhances sleep
- relieves anxiety
- relieves stress
- soothes body and mind

SPRUCE

has a middle note with a woody scent that is fresh with a slight hint of fruit. It is calming to the nervous system and encourages communication. It comes from an evergreen that grows wild in both Canada and Europe.

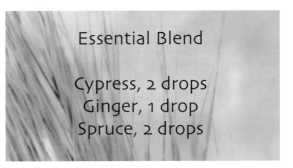

Essential Blend

Cypress, 2 drops
Ginger, 1 drop
Spruce, 2 drops

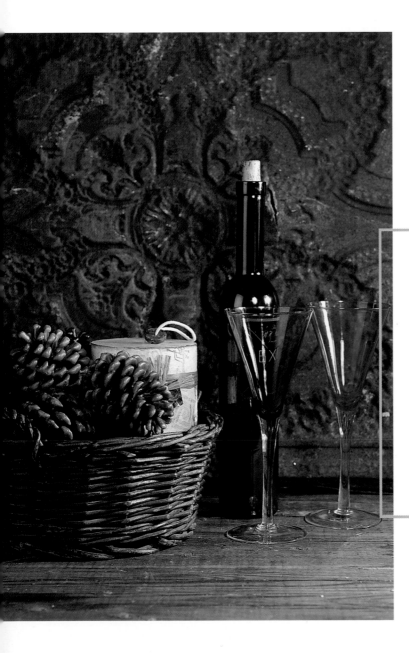

SPRUCE IT UP

dipping pot
double boiler
dyes: green, purple
essential oils: cypress, ginger, spruce
kitchen scale
metal slotted spoon
pinecones: medium-sized
taper-blend wax
thermometer
waxed paper

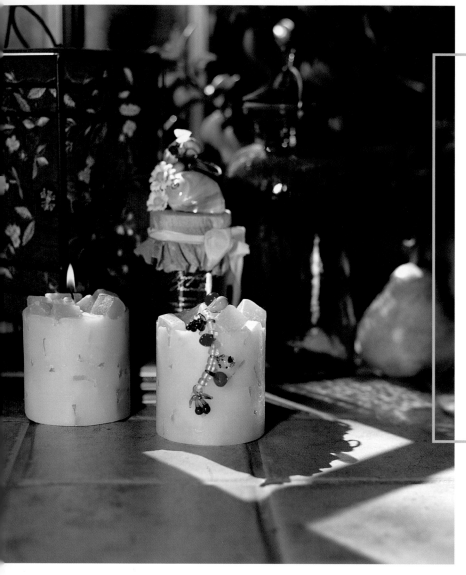

LEMON LIGHT

double boiler
essential oils: lavender, lemon,
    lemongrass
fruit beads
kitchen scale
metal pouring pot
metal skewer
mold: 3"-diameter round pillar
mold release
mold sealer
mold-blend wax
primed wick: square-braided
scissors
thermometer
wax chunks: yellow

Essential Blend

Lavender, 1 drop
Lemon, 3 drops
Lemongrass, 1 drop

LEMON has a top note with a fresh citrus scent. The refreshing scent is cooling, balancing, improves mental clarity, and helps to relieve fatigue. This essential oil is extracted from the peel and lends a fresh scent to any blend. Lemon can be antiseptic and is good for building up the immune system.

chunk candle

1 Using double boiler, melt wax.

2 Using mold release, lightly coat inside of candle mold.

3 Determine wick length and add 3". Cut wick and thread through hole in bottom of mold and secure.

4 Position yellow wax chunks in candle mold as desired.

5 Pour melted wax into metal pouring pot.

6 Add essential blend to melted wax.

7 Pour melted wax into mold until 90% full. Allow wax to set.

8 Place additional wax chunks into mold, allowing them to protrude from melted wax. Allow wax to set.

9 Tip mold upside down and remove candle.

10 Trim wick at bottom of candle, allowing top of wick to remain long enough to thread fruit beads for decoration. Note: Fruit beads must be removed and wick trimmed before burning.

Lemon blends well with:
  cedarwood
  eucalyptus
  fennel
  juniper
  ylang-ylang

Other benefits and uses for lemon:
  enhances mood
  purifies body and mind

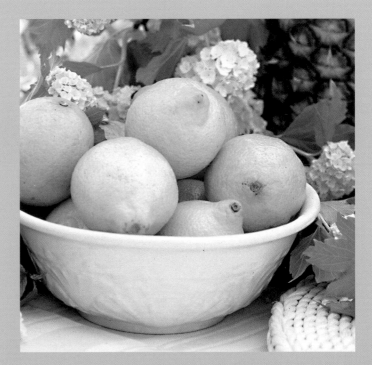

BAYBERRY WAX

has a soothing and fragrant aroma that does not require the addition of other scents. The wax is extracted by boiling the berries and skimming off the wax. Bayberry is not a true essential oil and it is usually found as a manmade fragrance or a bayberry essence in a carrier oil at best. The berries and bark of the bayberry bush have the medicinal properties of being an astringent, aiding intestinal problems and jaundice.

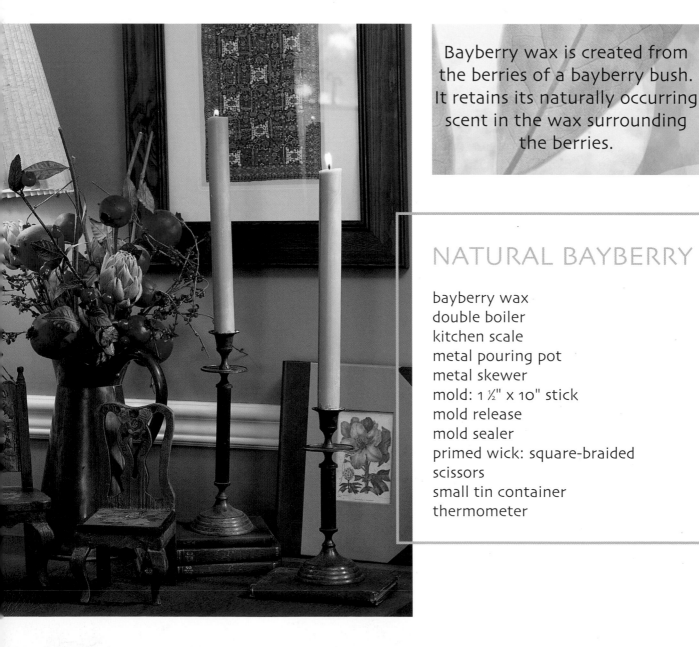

Bayberry wax is created from the berries of a bayberry bush. It retains its naturally occurring scent in the wax surrounding the berries.

NATURAL BAYBERRY

bayberry wax
double boiler
kitchen scale
metal pouring pot
metal skewer
mold: 1 ½" x 10" stick
mold release
mold sealer
primed wick: square-braided
scissors
small tin container
thermometer

bayberry pillars

1

Using double boiler, melt wax.

2

Using mold release, lightly coat inside of mold.

3

Cut wick to appropriate length and thread through hole in bottom of mold and secure.

4

Pour melted wax into metal pouring pot.

5

Pour melted wax into mold until 90% full. Pour excess wax into tin container. Allow wax to set.

6

Remelt excess wax and fill indentation. Allow wax to set.

7

Tip mold upside down and remove candle.

8

Trim wick at top and bottom of candle.

tips

Bayberry wax may be combined with beeswax in a ratio of 8:2.

It has been a tradition since colonial days to burn a bayberry candle down to a nub on New Year's Eve to bring health and happiness for the coming year.

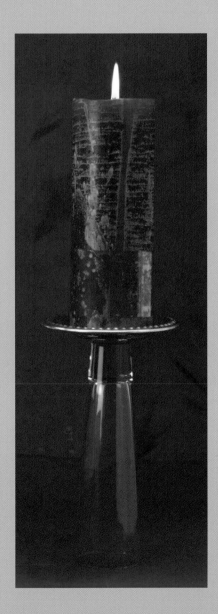

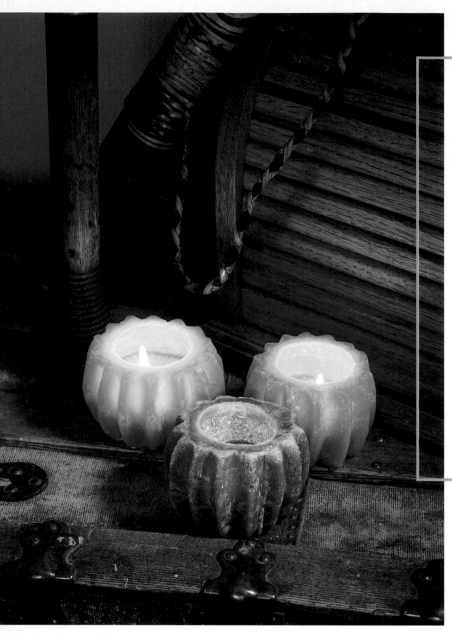

BALMY BASIL

aluminum foil
double boiler
dye: gold
electric skillet
essential oils: basil, lavender, rosemary
funnel
kitchen scale
metal pouring pot
mold: round fluted (large enough for
　　yogurt container to sit with
　　¼"–½" gap around outside
mold release
mold-blend wax
plastic yogurt container
small tin container
thermometer
unscented votive: gold

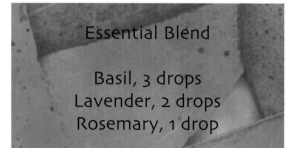

Essential Blend

Basil, 3 drops
Lavender, 2 drops
Rosemary, 1 drop

BASIL has a top note that is herbaceous in scent. It is stimulating to the mind and cheering to the soul. It helps to increase concentration and chases away the blues and mental fatigue. Like many herbs, it originally came from Asia and was highly favored by the Greeks.

candle lanterns

1 Using double boiler, melt wax.

2 Using mold release, lightly coat inside of mold and outside of yogurt container.

3 Pour melted wax into metal pouring pot.

4 Add dye to melted wax.

5 Pour ½" of melted wax into bottom of mold. Allow wax to set.

6 Place yogurt container into mold and center. Fill yogurt container with cold water.

7 Using funnel, pour melted wax between outside edge of yogurt container and inside of mold until 90% full. Pour excess wax into tin container. Allow wax to set.

8 Remelt excess wax and fill indentation if necessary. Allow wax to set.

9 Tip mold upside down and remove candle.

10 Line skillet with aluminum foil. Heat skillet and place top side of candle onto foil to smooth candle edge.

11 Scent gold votive candle with essential blend. See Using Purchased Candles on pages 25–26. Note: A votive candle could be made and scented with essential blend.

12 Place votive inside of hurricane.

tip

Hurricane can also be scented with essential blend.

Basil blends well with:
    bergamot
    geranium
    lavender

Other benefits and uses for basil:
    antidepressant
    purifies body and mind
    revitalizes body

SIGHT

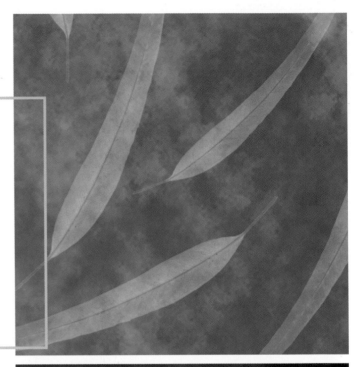

METAL

Budgeting
Business
Controlled planning
Financial stability
Leadership skills
Organizational skills
Project completion

Of the five senses sight has always been the most emphasized. We live in a visual society that is stimulated by all that it sees. One of the major elements in what we see is COLOR. To further awaken your senses, surround yourself with vibrant and invigorating primary colors of red, yellow, and blue. Red excites, stimulates, attracts energy, and increases metabolism. It is desire and passion. Yellow makes a strong statement; it is warm, cheerful, and the color of dance. Blue is a natural color; it calms, refreshes, and relaxes. It is also a chameleon—dark blue is strong and proud, while light blue is soft and kind. Metals of all finishes also stimulate the senses. Place your candles in shiny gold or silver candleholders— this adds a touch of opulent wealth.

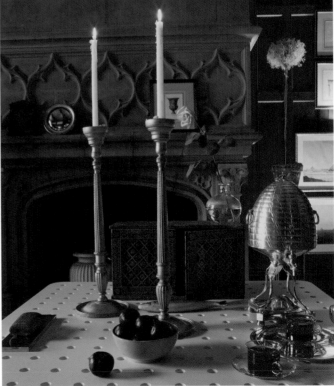

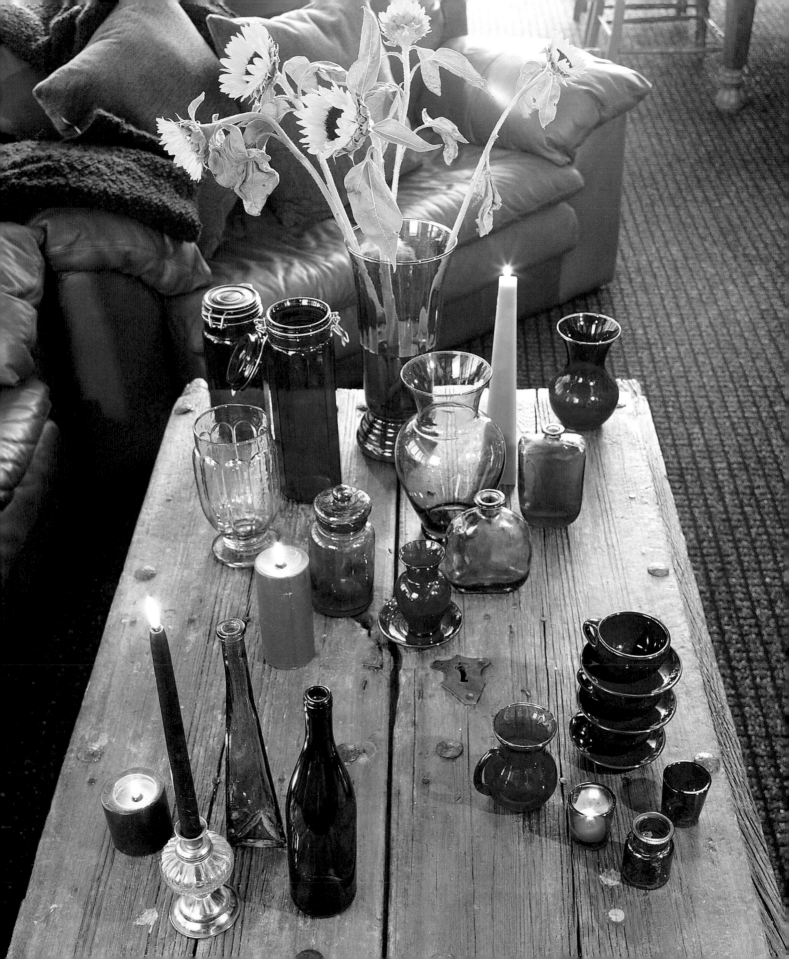

TURN IT ON

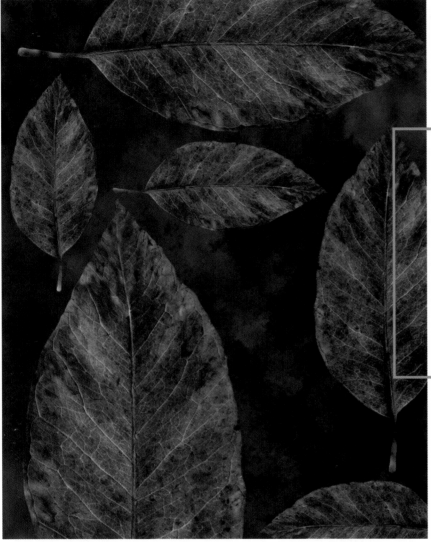

For the five senses to kindle feelings of love and romance, place your candles in a darkened room with hints of black satin and red silk, feast on champagne and strawberries, and listen to the sounds of love.

Ignite romance and burning desire. . . . The plant world is rich with aphrodisiac substances—this has been known since antiquity. However, reactions can be quite diverse. While one might melt away smelling the rich bouquet of patchouli, it might be perceived as too intense by someone else. Rose and jasmine, while queens amongst the scents, are often considered "too sweet", especially by men. If you are planning to create a surprise for your special someone, make certain you know their favorites first.

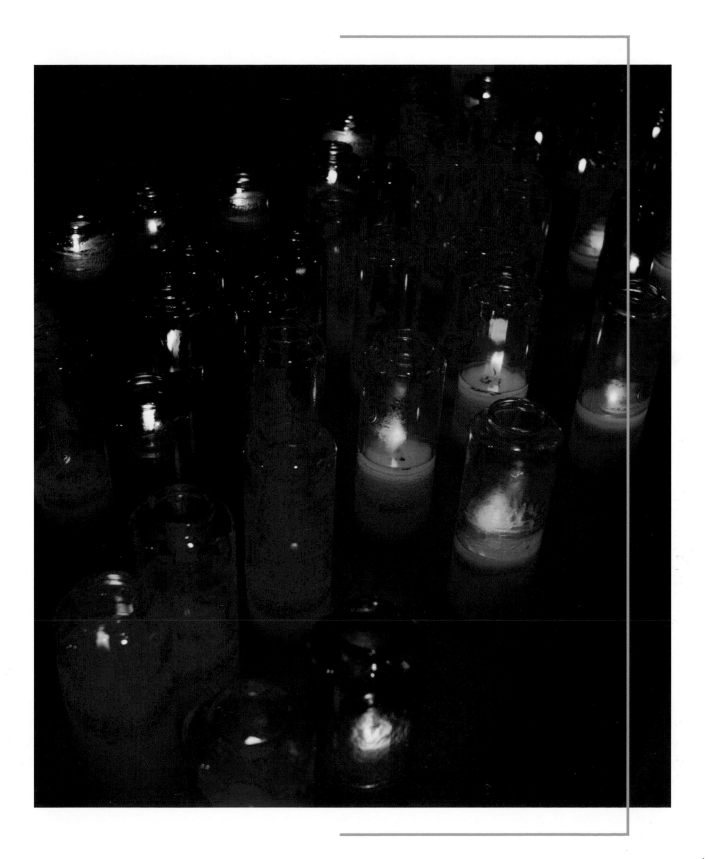

SANDALWOOD SCENT

dipping vat
double boiler
dowel
dye: amber
essential oils: cedarwood, jasmine,
    sandalwood
kitchen scale
paring knife
scissors
taper-blend wax
thermometer
wick: flat-braided

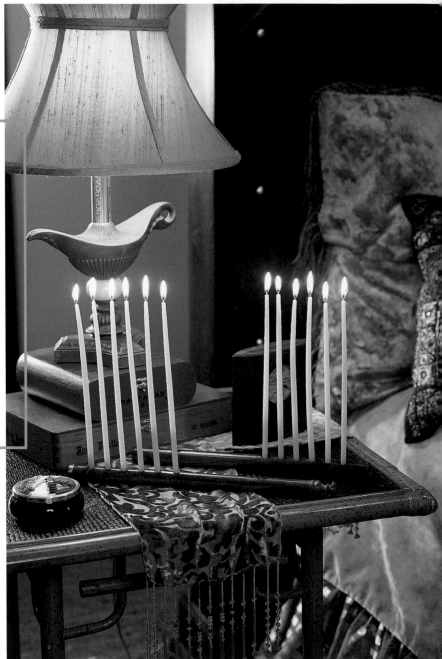

Essential Blend

Cedarwood, 3 drops
Jasmine, 1 drop
Sandalwood, 3 drops

SANDALWOOD has a base note with a fragrant yet
delicate aroma that has hints of both floral and woody scents. It is an aphrodisiac and blends well
with other essential oils that have this characteristic. Sandalwood's rich fragrance heightens
mental clarity and concentration, and is highly prized in incense. It has had many uses throughout the past; the Egyptians used it for embalming, it has been used as a building material for
temples, and it is favored in meditation because of the harmony it brings to the soul.

skinny tapers

1 Using double boiler, melt wax to 158°F.

2 Cut wick to desired height of candle times two plus 2".

3 Pour melted wax into dipping vat.

4 Add amber dye to melted wax.

5 Add essential blend to melted wax.

6 Fold wick in half and place wick over dowel. Dip the two ends into melted wax. Allow wicks to remain in wax for sixty seconds. Remove from wax, making certain that ends do not touch.

7 Hold candles over melted wax and allow wax to harden. Repeat dipping. After 3–4 dippings, use fingers and straighten wick and candle as necessary.

8 Repeat dipping. Note: Dip the candle a little shorter than full length each time to taper end. Using paring knife, trim bottoms of candles flat several times during the dipping process.

9 Repeat dipping process until desired thickness is achieved.

10 Trim bottoms of candles flat.

11 Trim wick at top and bottom of candles.

Sandalwood blends well with:
  frankincense
  lavender
  rose
  ylang-ylang

Other benefits and uses for sandalwood:
  antidepressant
  relieves stress
  soothes body and mind

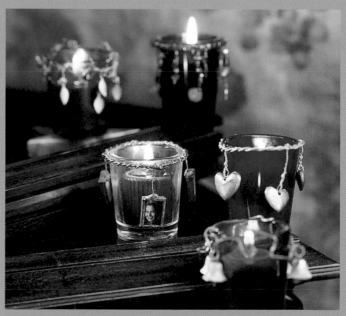

heart-carved candle

1 Place mold into freezer for 30 minutes. Note: The chilled mold will create a rustic look on outside of candle.

2 Using double boiler, melt wax.

3 Using mold release, lightly coat inside of mold.

4 Cut wick to appropriate length and thread through hole in bottom of mold and secure.

5 Pour melted wax into metal pouring pot.

6 Add red dye to melted wax.

7 Add essential blend to melted wax.

8 Pour melted wax into chilled mold until 90% full. Pour excess wax into tin container. Allow wax to set.

9 Remelt excess wax and fill indentation. Allow wax to set.

10 Tip mold upside down and remove candle.

11 Using craft knife, carve various sized hearts onto outside of candle in random pattern. Using flat edge of carving tool, carefully scrape wax from inside of heart shape. Note: A soft cloth may be used to buff out scrape marks from inside of hearts.

12 Trim wick at top and bottom of candle.

Jasmine blends well with:
    cedarwood
    neroli
    sandalwood

Other benefits and uses for jasmine:
    antidepressant
    reduces muscle tension
    soothes body and mind

PLEASANT JASMINE

craft carving tool or screwdriver
    with flat edge
craft knife
double boiler
dye: red
essential oils: jasmine, rose,
    ylang-ylang
kitchen scale
metal pouring pot
metal skewer
mold: round pillar
mold release
mold sealer
mold-blend wax
primed wick: square-braided
scissors
small tin container
thermometer

Essential Blend

Jasmine, 2 drops
Rose, 1 drop
Ylang-ylang, 1 drop

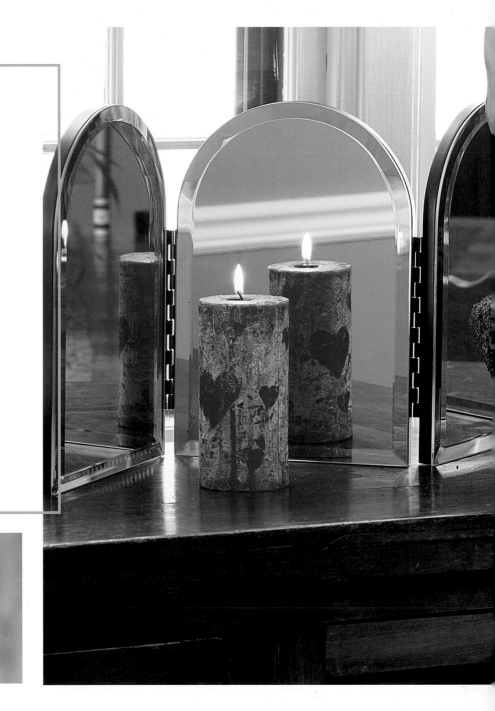

JASMINE
has a middle note and its sweet floral scent is renowned as an aphrodisiac. It is believed that jasmine can reawaken passions—allowing the heart to feel—reuniting love. In India, this fragrant flower has been called "Queen of the Night." It is warming to the emotions and restores positive feelings.

PATCHOULI

has a base note with an intense exotic musky scent that is best used in small amounts since it can be overpowering. Its sensual fragrance makes it a popular choice as an aphrodisiac. Patchouli tends to evoke extreme responses as well as allowing one to release pent-up emotions.

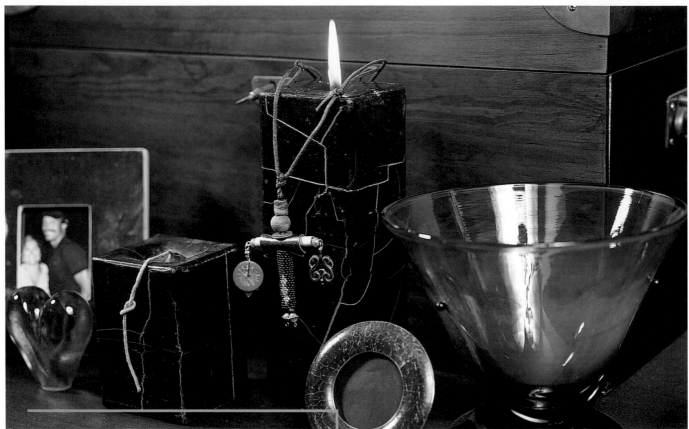

PURE PATCHOULI

candle paint: dark brown
dipping vat
double boiler
dye: brown
essential oils: patchouli, rose,
    sandalwood
kitchen scale
metal pouring pot
opaque crystals
sponge paintbrush
taper-blend wax
thermometer
unscented square pillar candle: tan
waxed paper

Essential Blend

Patchouli, 5 drops
Rose, 2 drops
Sandalwood, 2 drops

cracked candle

1 Using double boiler, melt wax. Add opaque crystals, following manufacturer's directions.

2 Scent tan pillar candle with essential blend. See Using Purchased Candles on pages 25–26. Note: A square pillar candle could be made and scented with essential blend.

3 Place pillar candle in freezer for 1–2 hours.

4 Paint cold candle with brown candle paint. Allow paint to dry until tacky, then return candle to freezer for 15–20 minutes.

5 Add dye to melted wax. Melted wax should be dyed as dark brown as possible.

6 Pour melted wax into dipping vat.

7 Holding candle by wick, dip candle into dipping pot in one smooth motion. Repeat dipping two additional times. Place on waxed paper.

8 Return candle to freezer for 1–2 hours. Note: The longer the candle is left in the freezer, the more cracks will appear.

9 Allow candle to warm to room temperature. Using fingers, carefully press outside of candle to smooth out any air bubbles.

tip

Dipping wax may also be scented with essential blend.

Patchouli blends well with:
- basil
- bergamot
- geranium
- jasmine
- lemon
- pine
- ylang-ylang

Other benefits and uses for patchouli:
- antidepressant
- enhances sleep
- soothes body and mind
- uplifting

floating snowflake candle

1 Using double boiler, melt wax.

2 Using mold release, lightly coat inside of mold.

3 Cut wick 1" longer than mold depth.

4 Pour melted wax into metal pouring pot.

5 Add essential blend to melted wax.

6 Pour melted wax into mold until 90% full. Pour excess wax into tin container. Allow wax to set.

7 Remelt excess wax and fill indentation. Allow wax to set.

8 Tip mold upside down and remove candle.

9 Dip wicking needle into hot water to warm needle. Pierce hole through center of candle large enough for wick to pass through. Note: Hole should not be so large that wick will slide out.

10 Trim or pull wick flush with bottom of candle.

11 Line electric skillet with aluminum foil. Heat electric skillet and place bottom side of candle onto foil to smooth candle base and seal wick into wax. Note: Make certain that wick is thoroughly sealed to prevent water from getting into candle.

12 Sprinkle warm candle with glitter and trim top of wick.

tip

Use muffin tins and tiny tart pans as molds for floating candles.

Ylang-ylang blends well with:
- bergamot
- jasmine
- neroli
- orange
- sandalwood

Other benefits and uses for ylang-ylang:
- antidepressant
- calms anger and frustration
- relieves anxiety
- relieves stress

YLANG-YLANG

has a middle note with a floral, yet spicy fragrance commonly used in perfumes. It has a scent that is erotic and very feminine. It relieves sexual anxiety and is emotionally warming. It is best to use ylang-ylang sparingly and in a blend since it can be too sweet and overuse can cause headaches and nausea.

Essential Blend

Black pepper, 1 drop
Mandarin orange, 2 drops
Ylang-ylang, 2 drops

YLANG-YLANG DREAM

aluminum foil
double boiler
electric skillet
essential oils: black pepper,
    mandarin orange, ylang-ylang
glitter
kitchen scale
metal pouring pot
mold: snowflake
mold release
mold-blend wax
primed wick: square-braided
scissors
small tin container
thermometer
wicking needle

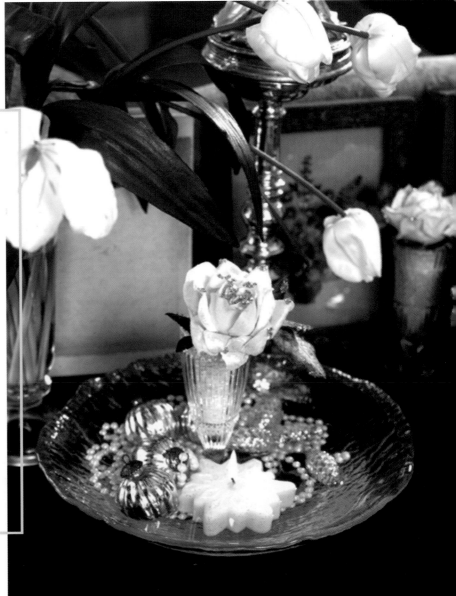

SMELL

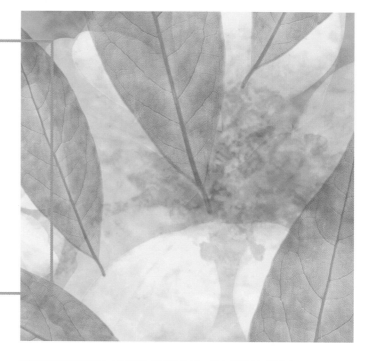

FIRE

Celebration
Expression
Fame
Mental stimulation
New ideas
Passion
Sociability
Spontaneity

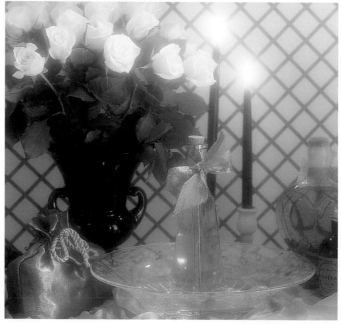

Nothing is more memorable than a favored scent. It can be natural or man-made. It can change a mood or create one. It is as individual as the person. It is as important to the overall human experience as any of the other stimulants to the other four senses. To awaken your senses of romance and desire, burn a candle that evokes passion, smells enticing, and promotes intimacy. You should choose a scent that is liked by both you and your partner. For some, the need to avoid heavy scents is replaced with the smell of fresh air and newly washed linens. Oils can be used not only in candles but rubbed on the body or diluted and gently sprayed onto the bedding.

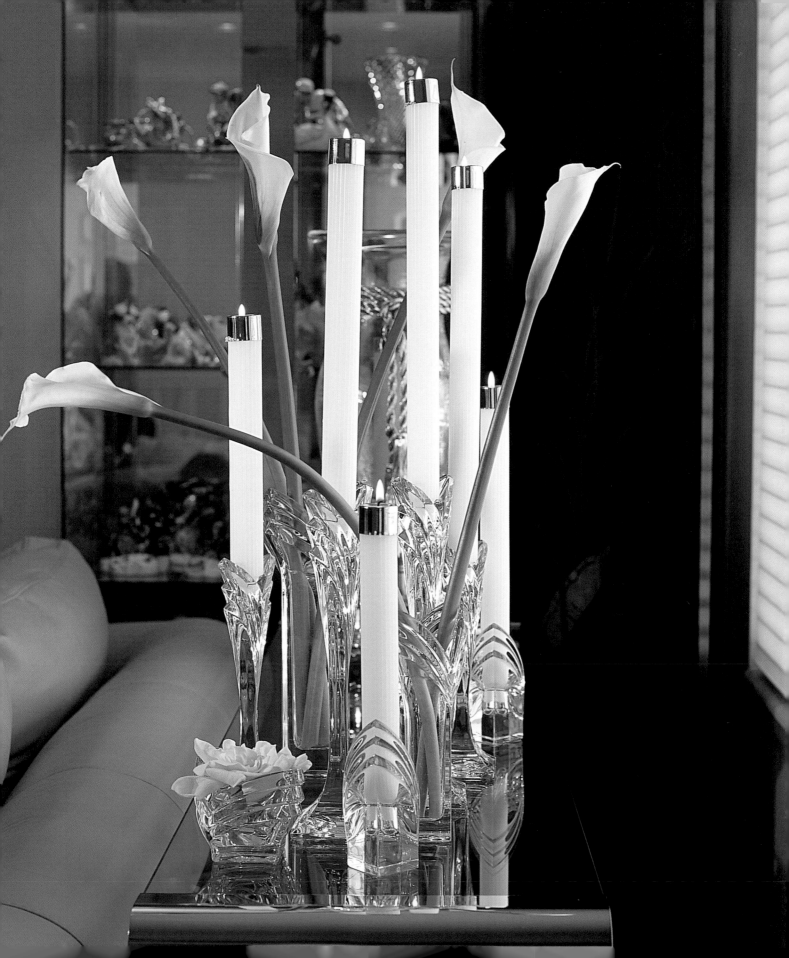

CELEBRATE

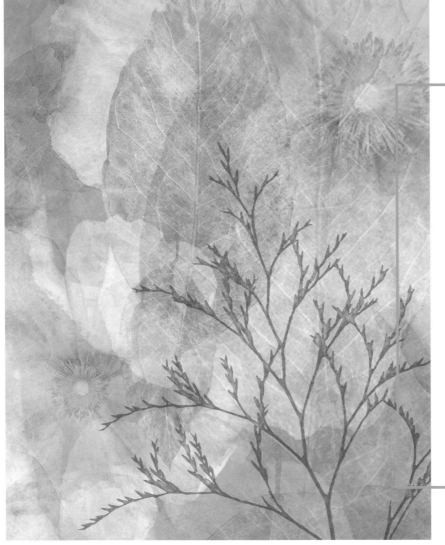

Add everything special to a celebration by giving small gifts to all of the senses. When your family and guests arrive, let them see party decorations of paper streamers and balloons in bright colors. Let them smell clove or cinnamon, let them eat cake and decadent sweets, let them open presents, and let them listen to the sounds of laughter.

Celebration times illuminated. . . . Whatever the occasion, aromatic candles add a spark to every event. Inspire your guests and create feelings of intimacy and splendor with the following settings. Candles always have been one of the best ways to express abundance. It does not take much to illuminate your event with an ocean of light.

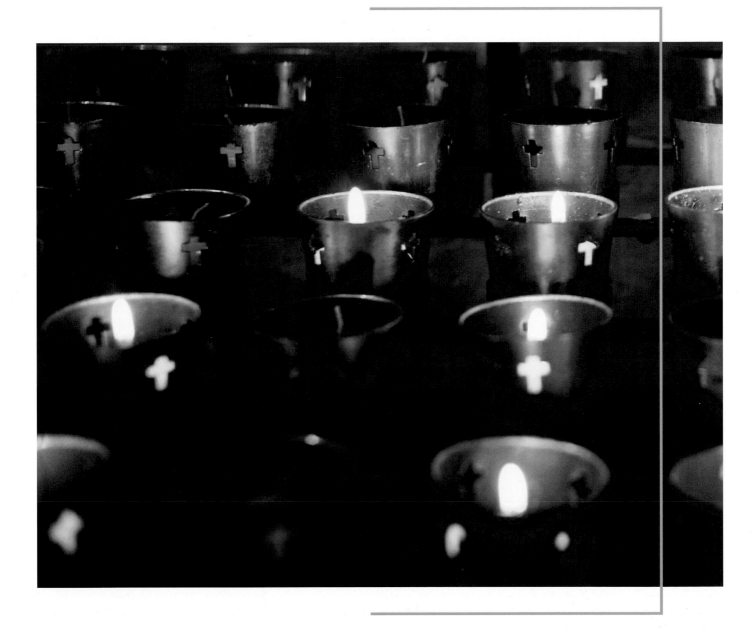

round floating candle

1 Using double boiler, melt wax.

2 Using mold release, lightly coat inside of mold.

3 Cut wick 1" longer than mold depth.

4 Pour melted wax into metal pouring pot.

5 Add essential blend to melted wax.

6 Add dye to melted wax.

7 Pour melted wax into mold until 90% full. Pour excess wax into tin container. Allow wax to set.

8 Remelt excess wax and fill indentation. Allow wax to set.

9 Tip mold upside down and remove candle.

10 Dip wicking needle into hot water to warm needle. Pierce hole through center of candle large enough for wick to pass through. Note: Hole should not be so large that wick will slide out.

11 Trim or pull wick flush with bottom of candle.

12 Line electric skillet with aluminum foil. Heat electric skillet and place bottom side of candle onto foil to smooth candle base and seal wick into wax. Note: Make certain that wick is thoroughly sealed to prevent water from getting into candle.

13 Trim top of wick.

tip

Fill vases or drinking glasses with plastic fruits or vegetables and water, then float candles above fruit.

Grapefruit blends well with:
- bergamot
- cedarwood
- chamomile
- lavender
- lemon
- rosemary

Other benefits and uses for grapefruit:
- reduces fatigue
- refreshes
- relieves stress

GRAPEFRUIT
has a top note with a refreshing and uplifting citrus fragrance. Grapefruit encourages clarity of thought and lightness of spirit. It can also aid in regulation of appetite and dismissing anxiety, as well as promoting a sense of well being and positive thinking.

Essential Blend

Grapefruit, 2 drops
Orange, 1 drop
Vanilla, 1 drop

SUNRISE GRAPEFRUIT

aluminum foil
double boiler
dye: yellow
electric skillet
essential oils: grapefruit, orange,
    vanilla
kitchen scale
metal pouring pot
mold: round floating
mold release
mold sealer
mold-blend wax
primed wick: square-braided
scissors
small tin container
thermometer
wicking needle

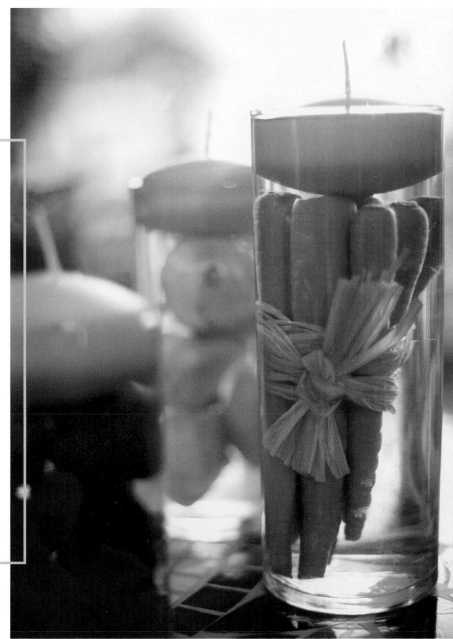

FRANKINCENSE

has a base note with a smoky, yet sweet and warming scent. It has been associated throughout the centuries with religious worship. It is distilled from the secreted beads of a gum-like resin. Frankincense encourages communication and elevates the mind and spirit. Its fragrance is commonly used in incense for meditation.

Essential Blend

Frankincense, 2 drops
Orange, 2 drops
Sandalwood, 1 drop

OLD FRANKINCENSE

acrylic paints: burgundy, purple
combing tool
double boiler
essential oils: frankincense, orange,
    sandalwood
hair dryer
kitchen scale
metal pouring pot
metal skewer
mold: tall square pillar
mold release
mold sealer
mold-blend wax
paintbrush
primed wick: square-braided
scissors
small tin container
soft cloth
thermometer

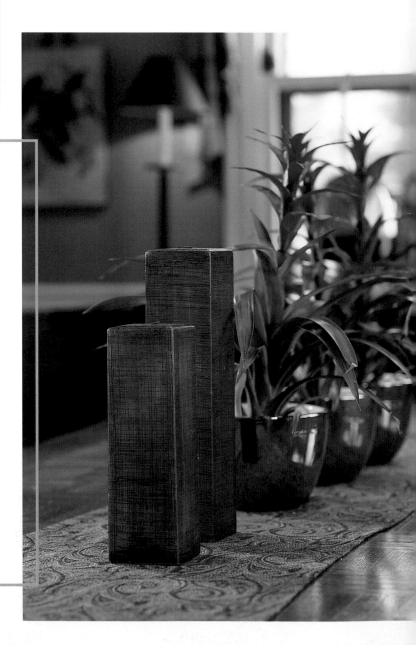

combed candles

1 Using double boiler, melt wax.

2 Using mold release, lightly coat inside of mold.

3 Cut wick to appropriate length and thread through hole in bottom of mold and secure.

4 Pour melted wax into metal pouring pot.

5 Add essential blend to melted wax.

6 Pour melted wax into mold until 90% full. Pour excess wax into tin container. Allow wax to set.

7 Remelt excess wax and fill indentation. Allow wax to set.

8 Tip mold upside down and remove candle.

9 Trim wick at top and bottom of candle.

10 Make second shorter candle, repeating Steps 1–9.

11 Using combing tool, drag comb down side of tallest candle to make fine grooves. Drag comb in on candle side to side so that grooves are going both directions.

12 Repeat Steps 11 for three remaining sides.

13 Repeat Steps 11–12 for shorter candle.

14 Apply burgundy paint to outside of tallest candle. Wipe off excess paint with soft cloth. Allow to dry.

15 Repeat Step 14 with purple paint on shorter candle.

16 Rub tallest candle with antiquing medium. Wipe off excess medium.

17 Repeat Step 16 for shorter candle.

double-molded candle

1 Using double boiler, melt wax.

2 Using mold release, lightly coat inside of mold.

3 Scent white pillar candle with essential blend. See Using Purchased Candles pages 25–26. Note: A round pillar candle could be made and scented with essential blend.

4 Center pillar candle in mold.

5 Arrange dried orange slices, pepper berries, leaves, and assorted foliage in mold.

6 Add dye to melted wax.

7 Pour melted wax into metal pouring pot.

8 Pour melted wax into mold over botanicals until 90% full. Pour excess wax into tin container.

9 Using dowel, rearrange any botanicals that may float out of place. Allow wax to set.

10 Remelt excess wax and fill indentation. Allow wax to set.

11 Tip mold upside down and remove candle.

12 Trim wick at top and bottom of candle.

Clove blends well with:
   cinnamon
   ginger
   peppermint
   rosemary

Other benefits and uses for clove:
   disinfects
   enhances mental clarity
   improves digestion
   loosens congestion
   reduces fatigue

SPICY CLOVE

assorted dried foliage
double boiler
dried orange slices
dye: gold
essential oils: clove, orange, vanilla
kitchen scale
large flat leaves
metal pouring pot
metal skewer
mold: large oval
mold release
mold sealer
mold-blend wax
pepper berries
primed wick: square-braided
scissors
small tin container
thermometer
unscented round pillar candle: white
    (smaller than mold)
wooden dowel

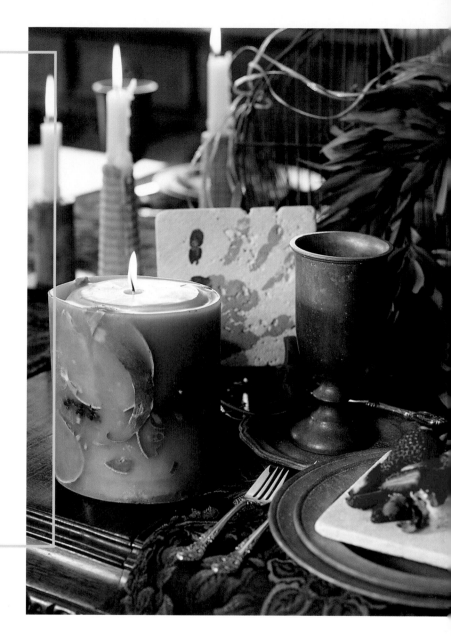

Essential Blend

Clove, 3 drops
Orange, 4 drops
Vanilla, 5 drops

CLOVE

has a base to middle note with a spicy scent. The fragrance is one that is warming and stimulating, as well as being considered an aphrodisiac. Clove should be used sparingly in any blend. The bud is used in cooking and potpourri. The oil is uplifting, relieves pain, and improves mental clarity and memory.

distressed pillars

1 Place mold into freezer for 30 minutes. Note: The chilled mold will create a rustic look on outside of candle.

2 Using double boiler, melt wax.

3 Using mold release, lightly coat inside of mold.

4 Cut wick to appropriate length and thread through hole in bottom of mold and secure.

5 Pour melted wax into metal pouring pot.

6 Add dye to melted wax. Note: Wax may be divided into separate containers and colored separately if more than one color of candle is being made.

7 Add essential blend to melted wax.

8 Pour melted wax into chilled mold until 90% full. Pour excess wax into tin container. Allow wax to set.

9 Trim wick at top and bottom of candle.

10 Tip mold upside down and remove candle.

11 Trim wick at top and bottom of candle.

Pine blends well with:
   grapefruit
   lemon
   myrrh
   neroli
   sandalwood
   vetiver

Other benefits and uses for pine:
   calms nerves
   enhances sleep
   relieves anxiety
   relieves stress

PINE

has a middle note with a fresh balsamic scent that may range from medium to strong. It is uplifting, energizing, and refreshing. Inhaling the vapors of pine will aid in breathing and has a purifying effect on the body

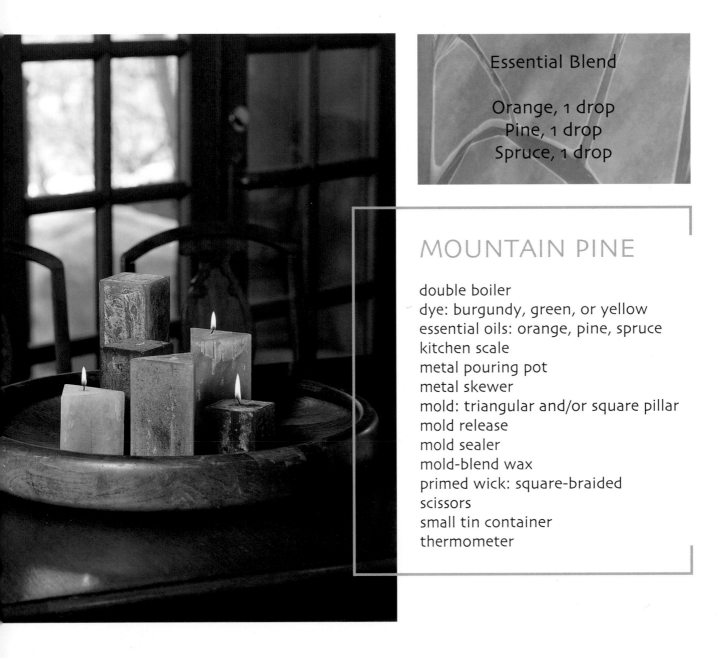

Essential Blend

Orange, 1 drop
Pine, 1 drop
Spruce, 1 drop

MOUNTAIN PINE

double boiler
dye: burgundy, green, or yellow
essential oils: orange, pine, spruce
kitchen scale
metal pouring pot
metal skewer
mold: triangular and/or square pillar
mold release
mold sealer
mold-blend wax
primed wick: square-braided
scissors
small tin container
thermometer

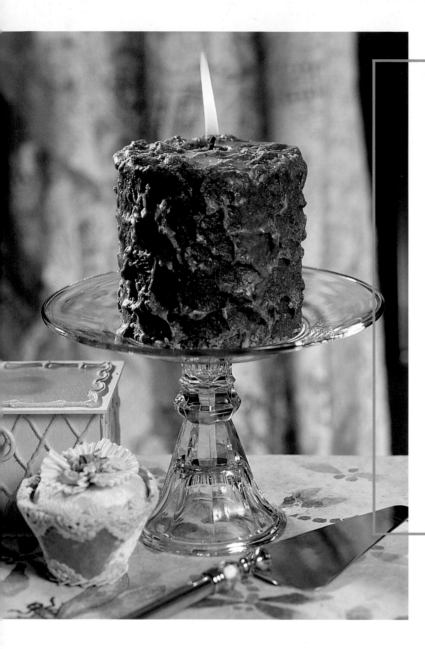

CINNAMON CANDY

double boiler
dye: red
essential oils: cedarwood, cinnamon,
    clove, orange
hair dryer
kitchen scale
metal fork
metal pouring pot
metal skewer
mold: 4"-diameter round pillar
mold release
mold sealer
mold-blend wax: enough for mold
    plus ½ as much more for
    whipping
primed wick: square-braided
scissors
small tin container
spatula
thermometer

Essential Blend

Cedarwood, 4 drops
Cinnamon, 1 drop
Clove, 1 drop
Orange, 3 drops

CINNAMON has a middle note and a rich, warming, spicy
scent that brings back memories of the holidays and smells wafting from the kitchen. It is
stimulating, strengthening, and warming to the mind, spirit, and body. It can banish feelings of
isolation and purify the air in a room.

frosted cake candle

1 Using double boiler, melt wax.

2 Using mold release, lightly coat inside of mold.

3 Cut wick to appropriate length and thread through hole in bottom of mold and secure.

4 Pour melted wax into pouring pot.

5 Add dye to melted wax.

6 Add essential blend to melted wax. Note: Reserve additional wax for whipping.

7 Pour melted wax into mold until 90% full. Pour excess wax into tin container. Allow wax to set.

8 Remelt excess wax and fill indentation. Allow wax to set.

9 Tip mold upside down and remove candle.

10 Allow reserved melted wax to cool until thin film appears on wax surface.

11 Using fork, whip wax until thick and foamy. Note: It may take 5–10 minutes to whip.

12 Warm sides of pillar candle with hair dryer.

13 Using spatula, apply a thick coat of wax to top and sides of candle. Note: Begin in one spot and cover that area completely before moving on to the next.

14 Trim wick at top and bottom of candle.

Cinnamon blends well with:
  coriander
  jasmine
  lemon
  sandalwood
  ylang-ylang

Other benefits and uses for cinnamon:
  aphrodisiac
  enhances mental clarity
  improves digestion
  reduces pain
  stimulates circulation

CARDAMOM CRAZE

decoupage medium
double boiler
dye: brown
essential oils: cardamom, grapefruit,
    vanilla
gold leaf
gold leafing medium
kitchen scale
metal pouring pot
metal skewer
mold: square
mold release
mold sealer
mold-blend wax
oriental-style newsprint or wrapping
    paper
paintbrush
primed wick: square-braided
ruler
scissors
small tin container
spatula
thermometer

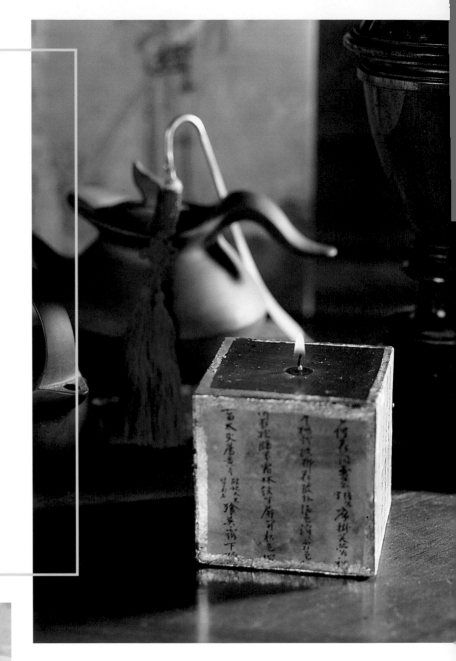

Essential Blend

Cardamom, 1 drop
Grapefruit, 2 drops
Vanilla, 1 drop

CARDAMOM has a middle note with a rich and warming spicy scent. It is uplifting and stimulating to the mind, reducing mental fatigue.

asian decoupaged candle

1 Using double boiler, melt wax.

2 Using mold release, lightly coat inside of mold.

3 Cut wick to appropriate length and thread through hole in bottom of mold and secure.

4 Pour melted wax into pouring pot.

5 Add dye to melted wax.

6 Add essential blend to melted wax.

7 Pour melted wax into mold until 90% full. Pour excess wax into tin container. Allow wax to set.

8 Remelt excess wax and fill indentation with melted wax. Allow wax to set.

9 Tip mold upside down and remove candle.

10 Trim wick at top and bottom of candle.

11 Measure sides of candle and cut four pieces of paper to those dimensions.

12 Apply decoupage medium to one side of candle. Place paper over decoupage medium and press to adhere to candle.

13 Apply decoupage medium over outside of paper and allow to dry. Repeat Steps 12–13 for three remaining sides.

14 Apply gold leafing medium and gold leaf to one side corner of candle, following manufacturer's instructions. Repeat for remaining corners, then top and bottom edges of candle.

tip

Decoupage fabric in place of paper to the sides of a candle.

Cardamom blends well with:
    cinnamon
    orange

Other benefits and uses for cardamom:
    enhances creativity
    improves digestion
    reduces pain

LEMONGRASS

has a top note with an herbaceous citrus fragrance. It is stimulating, revitalizing, and balancing to the nervous system. It can be used as a pick-me-up because of its mood-lightening properties. Lemongrass is a tall grass that has been used throughout the ages in Asia for flavoring food, and in India for medicinal purposes.

Essential Blend

Lavender, 2 drops
Lemongrass, 3 drops

GENTLE LEMONGRASS

cookie sheet
craft knife
double boiler
dye: white
essential oils: lavender, lemongrass
kitchen scale
metal pouring pot
metal skewer
mold release
mold sealer
mold-blend wax
primed wick: paper or metal core
scissors
small tin container
spatula
star cookie cutter
thermometer
wick tab
wicking needle

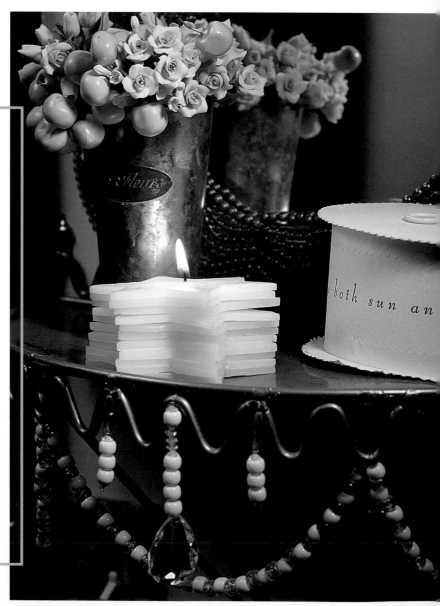

stacked-star candle

1 Using double boiler, melt wax.

2 Using mold release, lightly coat bottom of cookie sheet.

3 Pour melted wax into metal pouring pot.

4 Add dye to melted wax.

5 Add essential blend to melted wax.

6 Pour melted wax onto cookie sheet to the depth of ¼".

7 While sheet of wax is still warm, use cookie cutter to make star cutouts. Make certain to cut completely through wax to cookie sheet.

8 Using wicking needle, pierce hole in center of each star. Allow wax to set.

9 Using spatula, remove stars from cookie sheet.

10 Attach 12" of wick to wick tab.

11 Thread unattached end of wick onto wicking needle. Thread stars onto wick.

12 Trim wick at top.

Lemongrass blends well with:
   basil
   jasmine

Other benefits and uses for lemongrass:
   improves digestion
   reduces fatigue
   stimulates circulation

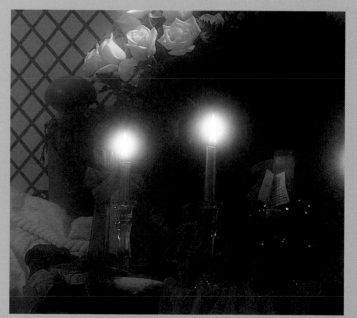

TASTE

WOOD

Activity
Ambition
Career
Concentration
Development
Industrious work
Initiative
Quick starts

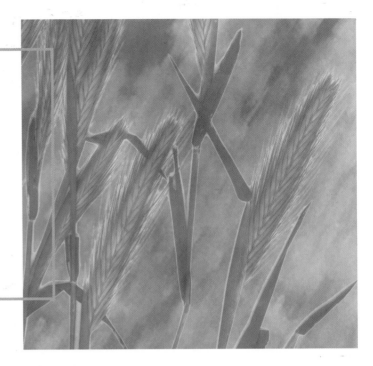

Taste is the most festive sense—the party sense. Think of taste, laughter, and food, and gatherings of people come to mind. When preparing to indulge the sense of taste remember—this is not the place to be conservative. The plates of food should be abundant, smell as good as they look, and look as good as they taste. Fine wines, the fresh fruits and vegetables of the season, main dishes seasoned with spices and herbs, and decadently rich desserts—all to be enjoyed throughout the evening. The table should be set with crystal that sparkles in the candlelight and china that is as translucent as the silk evening gowns on the ladies in attendance. This is an evening filled with accepted overindulgence.

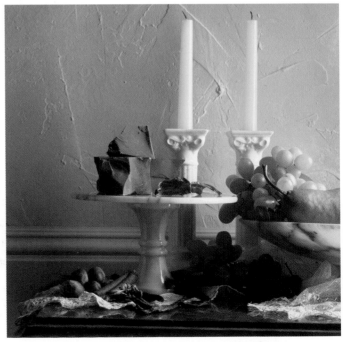

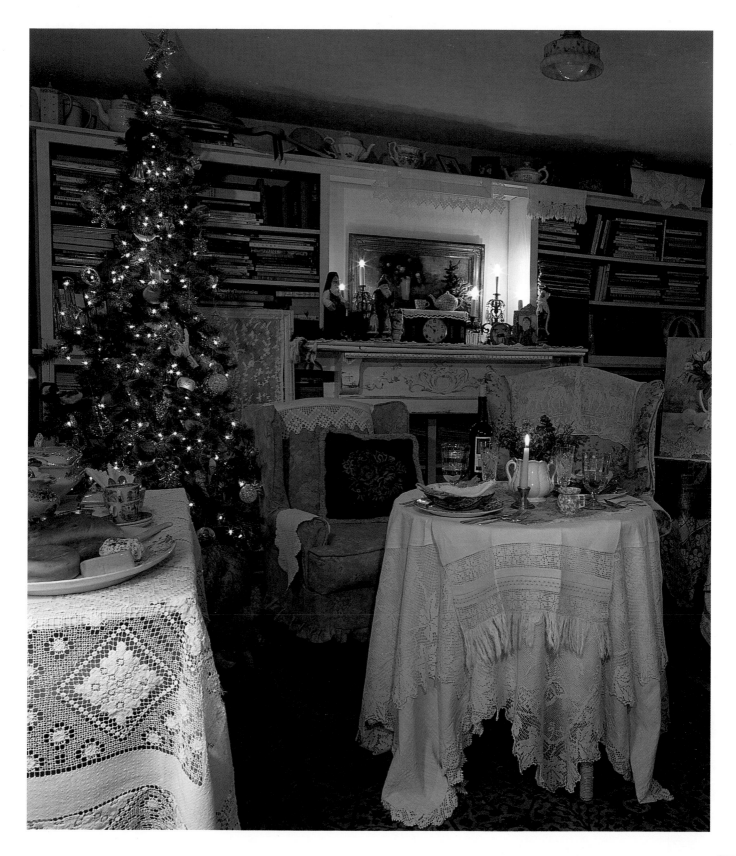

NURTURE WITH NATURE

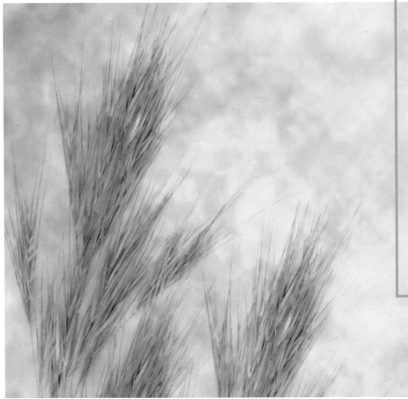

Again enlisting all the senses to renew yourself with the natural gifts of nature, sit in a pale room of green and enjoy its calming effects that help to enhance peace and contentment. Light candles that purify, eat fresh fruits and vegetables, lie under a down quilt, and listen to the soft sounds of silence.

. . . during renewal and sickness. The natural aromas of genuine essential oils are great friends for times of transition, whether that be a sickness, or a change in life that creates a need for nurturing. Inhaling these pure essences can fill you with peace, energy, and hope. Some of them also have positive effects on our respiratory and nervous system.

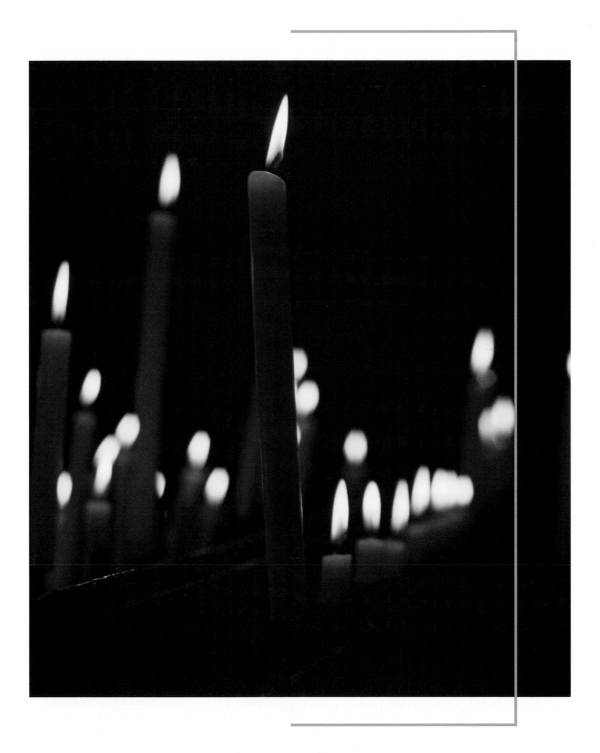

eucalyptus oil lamp

1

Arrange eucalyptus branches in decorative bottle as desired. Optional: Use floral wire to secure branches.

2

Place glass tube and wick into bottle and wire to branches to secure placement. Note: The tube should barely extend above the top of the bottle.

3

Add essential blend to lamp oil.

4

Pour oil into glass bottle. Adjust glass tube and wick if necessary.

tip

To prevent spills, a cork lid that fits the bottle could be drilled with a hole large enough for the tube to pass through.

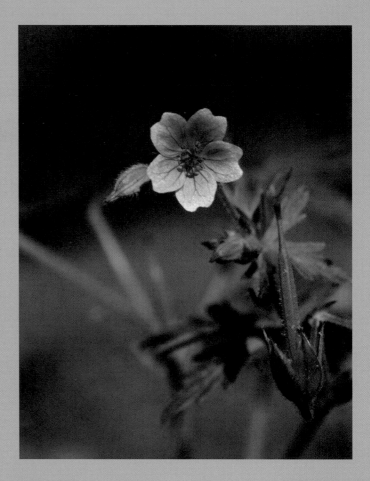

Eucalyptus blends well with:
> geranium
> juniper
> lemongrass
> pine

Other benefits and uses for eucalyptus:
> heightens imagination
> purifies body and mind
> refreshing
> soothes body and mind

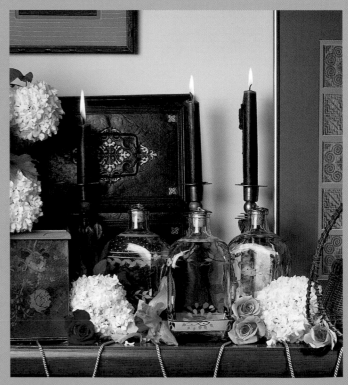

HEALING EUCALYPTUS

clear lamp oil
decorative bottle: clear, tall
essential oils: eucalyptus, lavender,
    lemon
eucalyptus branches
floral wire
glass tube with wick
wire cutters

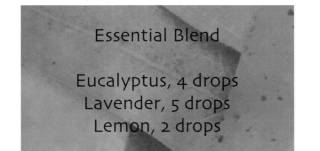

Essential Blend

Eucalyptus, 4 drops
Lavender, 5 drops
Lemon, 2 drops

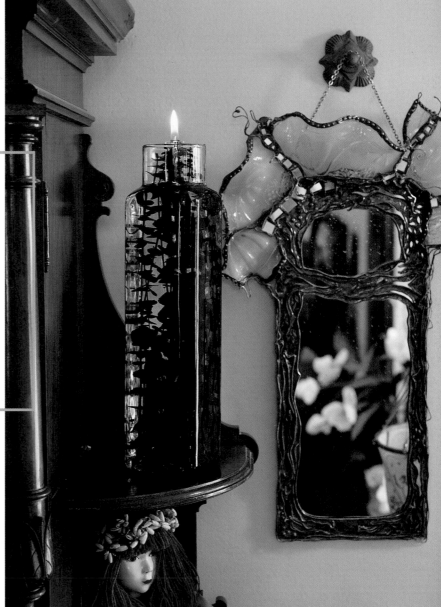

EUCALYPTUS has a top note with an herbaceous and fresh scent. Native to Australia, it is traditionally used for respiratory problems because it breaks up congestion and allows for deep breathing. Eucalyptus is also clearing to the mind, assisting one in concentration.

HELPFUL THYME

double boiler
dyes: red, yellow
essential oil: thyme
kitchen scale
metal pouring pot
metal skewer
mold: round pillar
mold release
mold sealer
mold-blend wax
primed wick: square-braided
scissors
small metal containers (2)
small tin container
thermometer

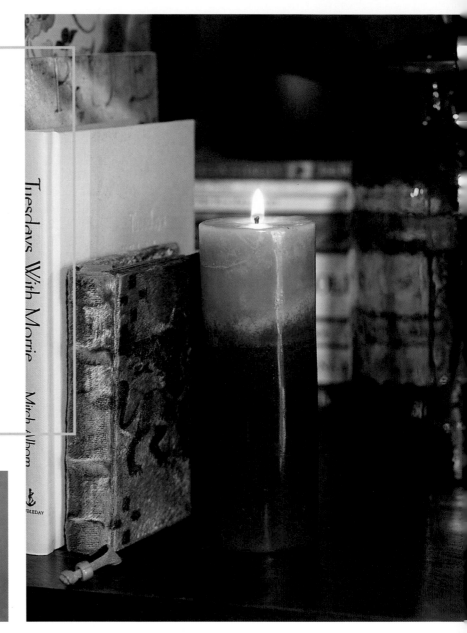

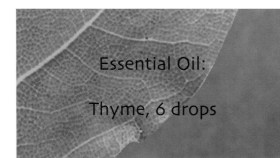

Essential Oil:

Thyme, 6 drops

THYME has a top note that is herbaceous and fresh. It warms and purifies

the body as well as relaxes tight muscles. Combined with elements of feng shui, thyme makes an ideal scent for nurturing communication and releasing judgment. The color red signifies fire. Fire promotes action and motivation. The color yellow signifies earth. Earth promotes security and stability.

fire and earth candle

1 Using double boiler, melt wax.

2 Using mold release, lightly coat inside of candle mold.

3 Cut wick to appropriate length and thread through hole in bottom of mold and secure.

4 Pour ⅔ of melted wax into metal pouring pot.

5 Add red dye to melted wax in metal pouring pot.

6 Divide essential oil into three parts and add two parts to melted wax in metal pouring pot.

7 Pour melted wax into mold until ⅔ full. Allow wax to set.

8 Pour remaining melted wax into metal pouring pot and add yellow dye.

9 Add remaining part of essential oil to melted wax as in Step 6.

10 Pour melted wax into mold until full. Allow wax to set.

11 Remelt any excess yellow wax and fill indentation. Allow wax to set.

12 Tip mold upside down and remove candle.

13 Trim wick at top and bottom of candle.

Thyme blends well with:
- lemon
- orange
- rosemary

Other benefits and uses for thyme:
- enhances mood
- improves digestion
- reduces pain

marbled candle

1 Using double boiler, melt wax.

2 Using mold release, lightly coat inside of mold.

3 Cut wick to appropriate length and thread through hole in bottom of mold and secure.

4 Add dye to melted wax.

5 Add essential blend to melted wax.

6 Pour melted wax into metal pouring pots, dividing wax equally. Place one pot into water in bottom half of double boiler to keep melted.

7 Allow wax in remaining pot to cool until light film forms. Using fork, whip the wax until foamy. Note: The whipped wax will be lighter in color than the melted wax.

8 Pour the melted and whipped waxes into mold simultaneously. Tap bottom of mold to settle wax. Allow wax to set.

9 Tip mold upside down and remove candle.

10 Trim wick at top and bottom of candle.

Rosemary blends well with:
- basil
- bergamot
- cedarwood
- lemon
- peppermint

Other benefits and uses for rosemary :
- increases energy
- reduces fatigue
- revitalizes body

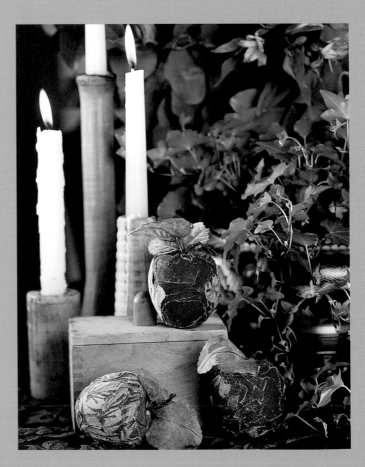

ROSEMARY

has a middle note with an herbaceous and camphorous scent. It is particularly good for mental exhaustion and lethargy. It improves mental clarity and memory as well as balancing mind and body. This evergreen shrub is also used for flavoring food and has antiseptic qualities when used in cleaning supplies.

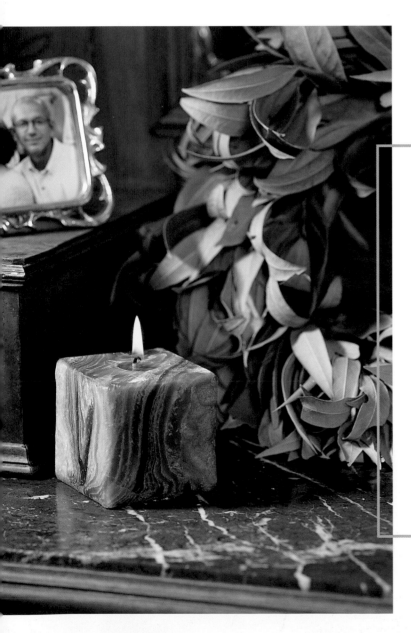

Essential Blend

Geranium, 1 drop
Juniper, 1 drop
Rosemary, 1 drop

ROSEMARY HERB

double boiler
dye: green
essential oils: geranium, juniper,
    rosemary
kitchen scale
metal fork
metal pouring pots (2)
metal skewer
mold: square
mold release
mold sealer
mold-blend wax
primed wick: square-braided
scissors
thermometer

pressed flower candle

1

Using double boiler, melt wax.

2

Scent white pillar candle with essential blend. See Using Purchased Candles on pages 25–26. Note: A round pillar can be made and scented with essential blend.

3

Using glue pen, attach flowers around outside of pillar candle as desired.

4

Pour melted wax into dipping pot.

5

Holding candle by wick, dip candle into dipping pot in one smooth motion. Place candle on waxed paper.

6

Carefully press down any flowers that protrude through wax. Allow wax to set.

tip

Dipping wax may also be scented with essential blend.

Geranium blends well with:
    chamomile
    citrus
    lemongrass
    rose

Other benefits and uses for geranium:
    disinfects
    enhances sleep
    loosens congestion
    reduces pain
    repels insects
    soothes and heals skin
    soothes muscle tension

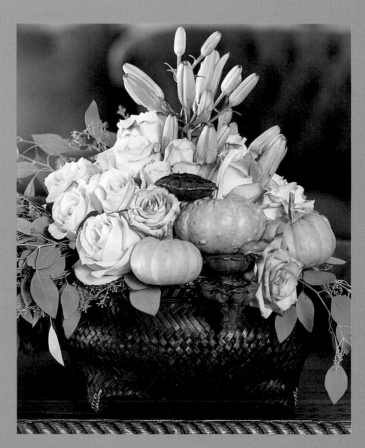

GERANIUM

has a middle note, with a delicate floral scent similar to that of a rose. It is a very popular scent in aromatherapy and a used in cosmetics as well as for flavoring food and drink. It can lessen pain and reduce inflammation. In small amounts, geranium can be calming and in large amounts, it may be stimulating.

Essential Blend

Bergamot, 2 drops
Geranium, 4 drops
Lavender, 1 drop

GERANIUM JOY

dipping vat
double boiler
essential oils: bergamot, geranium,
    lavender
glue pen
kitchen scale
metal pouring pot
paraffin wax
pressed flowers
thermometer
unscented round pillar candle: white
waxed paper

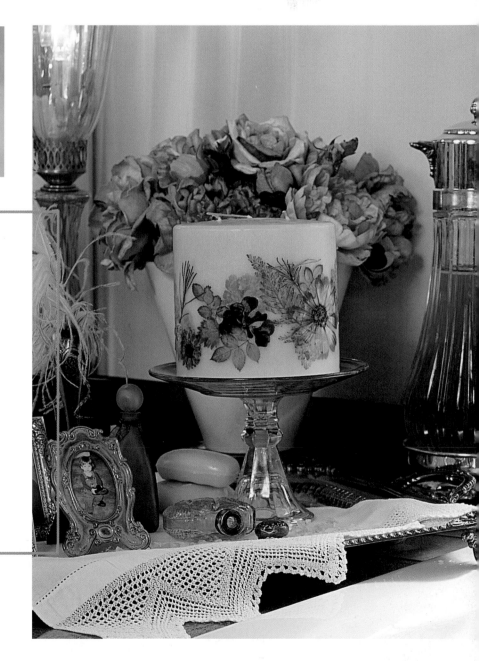

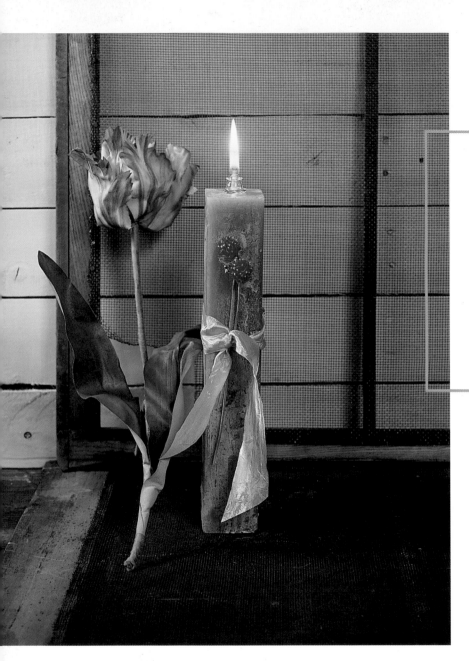

CLEANSING CAJEPUT

beige ribbon
drill and drill bit (size of glass vial)
dry flowers
essential oils: cajeput, lavender
glass vial with wick tubing
lamp oil
unscented pillar candle, sage-green
    (2" x 10")

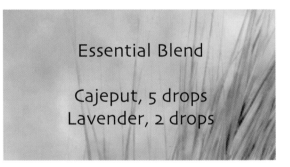

Essential Blend

Cajeput, 5 drops
Lavender, 2 drops

CAJEPUT has a top note with a strong and camphorous scent. It stimulates and energizes, making one's senses clear and alert. It is very effective in treating infection and cold symptoms. It has also been known to effectively ease the pain of headaches and other dull, aching pains.

glass vial candle

1 Carefully and slowly drill hole in center of candle to accommodate the length of glass vial. Note: Drilling quickly and without repeated pauses will cause candle wax to melt.

2 Insert glass vial into candle.

3 Add essential blend to lamp oil.

4 Pour oil into glass vial until 90% full.

5 Insert wick and tubing into vial.

6 Tie flowers to candle with ribbon.

Cajeput blends well with:
geranium
jasmine
lavender
orange

Other benefits and uses for cajeput:
antidepressant
relieves stress

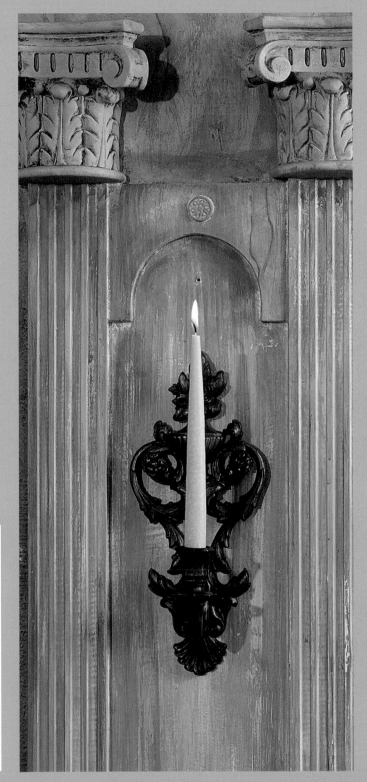

BERGAMOT

has a top note with a light citrus fragrance and a hint of floral. It has uplifting qualities, building one up emotionally and physically. Bergamot originates from the Mediterranean and is commonly used in eau de cologne and to flavor Earl Grey tea.

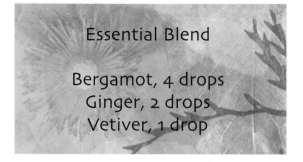

Essential Blend

Bergamot, 4 drops
Ginger, 2 drops
Vetiver, 1 drop

BERGAMOT BREEZE

butter knife
candle container
container-blend wax
cookie sheets (2)
craft knife
double boiler
dyes: orange, red
essential oils: bergamot, ginger,
    vetiver
hair dryer
kitchen scale
metal containers (2)
metal pouring pot
metal skewer
mold release
mold sealer
primed wick: paper or metal core
scissors
sharp kitchen knife
spatula
thermometer
wick tab
wicking needle

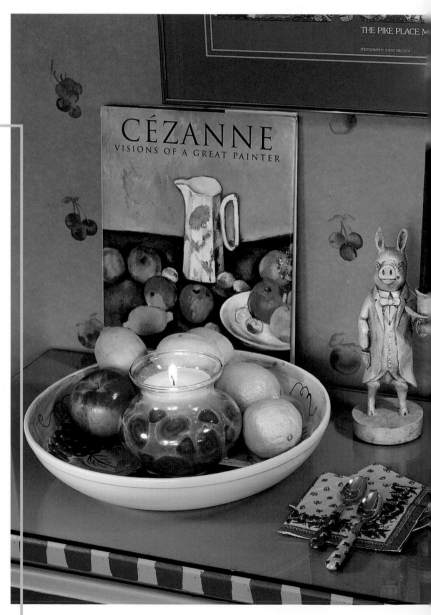

millifiore candle

1 Using double boiler, melt wax.

2 Using mold release, lightly coat bottom of cookie sheets.

3 Attach wick to wick tab.

4 Secure wick and tab to inside of container.

5 Pour melted wax into metal pouring pot.

6 Add essential blend to melted wax.

7 Pour some wax into each metal container, retaining the majority of wax for the container.

8 Add orange dye to melted wax in one container. Add red dye to melted wax in second container.

9 Pour orange melted wax onto one cookie sheet to the depth of ¼".

10 Pour red melted wax onto one cookie sheet to the depth of ⅛".

11 While sheets of wax are lukewarm, turn cookie sheets over and unmold wax onto a protected surface.

12 Using back of warm butter knife, cut wax into 1" x 4" pieces.

13 Stack one piece of orange wax onto one piece of red wax. Roll some of the wax pieces into a jelly-roll shape and others into triangular shapes. Note: Some rolls should have red on the outside and others should have orange.

14 Using sharp kitchen knife, slice wax rolls into ¼" slices.

15

Using hair dryer, warm outside of container and press wax shapes onto inside of container as desired.

16

When all slices have been placed onto sides of container, pour remaining uncolored melted wax into container until 90% full. Pour excess wax into tin container. Allow wax to set.

17

Remelt excess wax and fill indentation. Allow wax to set.

18

Trim wick at top of candle.

Bergamot blends well with:
- chamomile
- cypress
- jasmine
- lavender
- lemon
- neroli
- orange

Other benefits and uses for bergamot:
- enhances sleep
- improves healing
- relieves anxiety

SOUND

WATER

Affection
Conception
Independence
Inner growth
Sexuality
Sleep
Spirituality
Tranquility

If you want to hear the most beautiful sound you will ever hear, stand in your own backyard just as the sun is rising and listen to the music play. Close your eyes and listen to the quiet of life. Every sound is so clear, so pure, and so distinct. You can hear the birds celebrate the arrival of a new day, the wind gently whistling through the leaves on the trees; and you can almost hear the flowers open their buds to the warming rays of the sun while the grass drinks the morning dew. In these quiet, rare moments appreciate the sounds of nature—the sounds, the smells, the sights, and the gentle touch of nature.

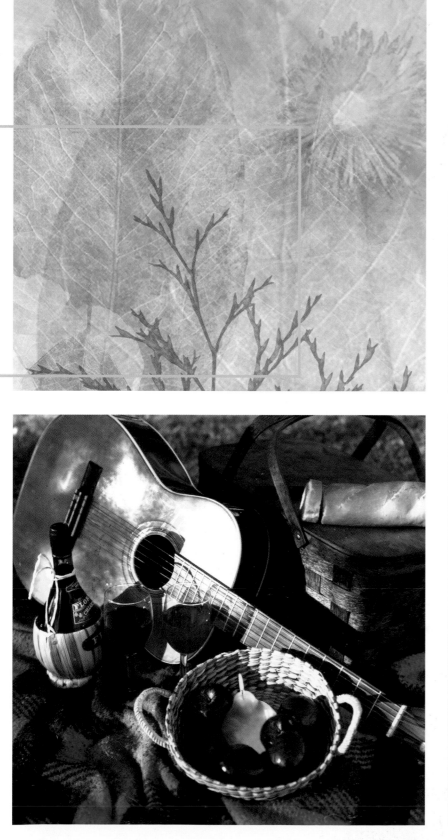
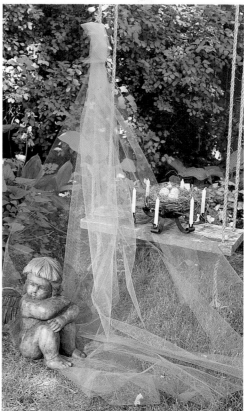
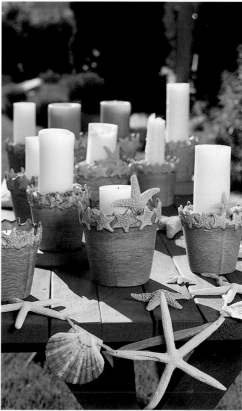

GENTLE SCENTS

All five senses can help enjoy a calm quiet afternoon. Gently soothe yourself to sleep with a cup of lemon-scented chamomile tea in a peaceful room of blue lit only with only candle light, surrounded by soft music, and tucked into clean cool crisp cotton sheets. It is here and now that you can drink deeply, dream, and believe.

Lullaby candles for calm and comfort. . . . Infusing your candle with the most soothing essential oils is a healthy and natural way to unwind and prepare for a good night's sleep. But wait . . . wait! You need to blow out the candle before you close your eyes! That is why I assembled so many ideas for container candles on these pages, just in case you simply cannot stay awake.

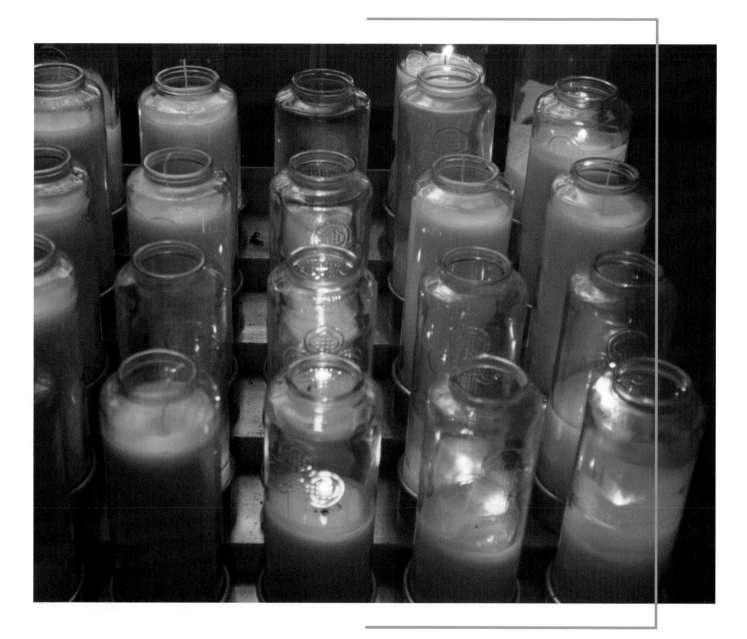

bamboo candle

1 Using hacksaw, cut bamboo into equal lengths ¼" shorter than mold height.

2 Using double boiler, melt wax.

3 Using mold release, lightly coat inside of mold.

4 Cut wick to appropriate length and thread through hole in bottom of mold and secure.

5 Line inside edge of mold with bamboo pieces. Secure bamboo pieces against inside edge of mold by placing hairpin through center of bamboo and over outside edge of mold.

6 Pour melted wax into metal pouring pot.

7 Add dye to melted wax.

8 Add essential blend to melted wax.

9 Pour melted wax into mold ¼" below the top edge of bamboo pieces. Pour excess wax into tin container. Allow wax to set.

10 Remove hair pins from bamboo pieces.

11 Remelt excess wax and fill indentation, allowing wax to flow onto top edge of bamboo pieces. Allow wax to set.

12 Tip mold upside down and remove candle.

13 Scrape off excess wax from around bamboo pieces.

14 Trim wick at top and bottom of candle.

Chamomile blends well with:
    cedarwood
    geranium
    melissa
    neroli
    rose

Other benefits and uses for chamomile:
    enhances sleep
    improves healing
    reduces inflammation
    refreshing
    soothes body and mind

CHAMOMILE

has a middle note with a mild herbaceous and slightly sweet fruity scent. It is gentle and has been used in a more traditional manner to soothe and calm small children as well as adults. It eases irritability, calms the mind, and encourages patience. It works well in sleep pillows for insomnia and baths to relax.

Essential Blend

Chamomile, 1 drop
Lavender, 3 drops
Vanilla, 2 drops

SMOOTH CHAMOMILE

bamboo: ⅜"–½" diameter
craft knife
double boiler
dye: green
essential oils: chamomile, lavender,
    vanilla
hair pins
kitchen scale
metal pouring pot
metal skewer
mold: round pillar
mold release
mold sealer
mold-blend wax
primed wick: square-braided
scissors
small hacksaw
small tin container
thermometer

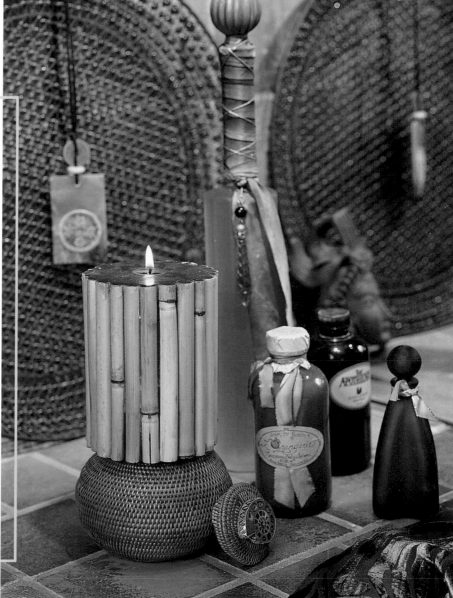

FRAGRANT ROSE

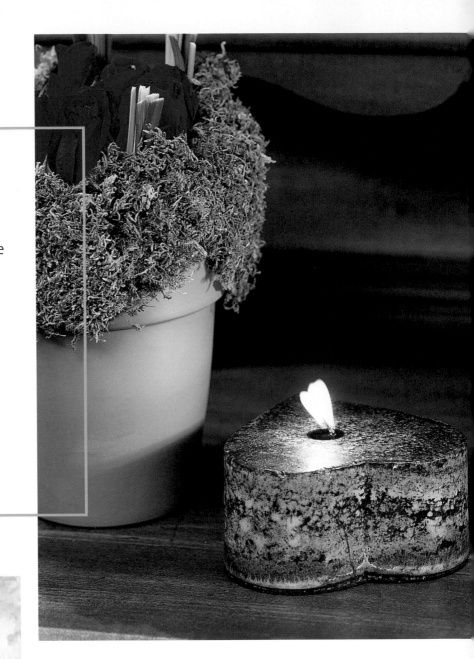

double boiler
dye: red
essential oils: lavender, orange, rose
kitchen scale
metal pouring pot
metal skewer
mold: large heart
mold release
mold sealer
mold-blend wax
primed wick: square-braided
scissors
small tin container
snowflake or mineral oil
thermometer

Essential Blend

Lavender, 2 drops
Orange, 2 drops
Rose, 3 drops

ROSE has a base note with a timeless and most popular floral scent. It has a sweet and gentle aroma that is purifying, uplifting, and calming. The rose is a symbol of love and compassion, and brings with it a feeling of bliss and harmony.

heart-shaped candle

1 Using double boiler, melt wax.

2 Using mold release, lightly coat inside of mold.

3 Cut wick to appropriate length and thread through hole in bottom of mold and secure.

4 Add snowflake oil, following manufacturer's directions. Note: If using mineral oil, add 2 tablespoons of mineral oil per pound of wax.

5 Pour melted wax into metal pouring pot.

6 Add dye to melted wax.

7 Add essential blend to melted wax.

8 Pour melted wax into mold until 90% full. Pour excess wax into tin container. Allow wax to set.

9 Remelt excess wax and fill indentation. Allow wax to set.

10 Tip mold upside down and remove candle.

11 Trim wick at top and bottom of candle.

tips

A high level of added essential oils can also create this snowflake effect which is called starburst or mottling.

Reducing the amount of snowflake or mineral oil will result in a slighter effect, while increasing the amount will result in stronger crystalline shapes.

Rose blends well with:
- geranium
- jasmine
- lavender
- neroli
- orange
- sandalwood
- ylang-ylang

Other benefits and uses for rose:
- antidepressant
- aphrodisiac
- refreshing

shell oil lamp

1

Arrange seashells and beach glass in jar as desired.

2

Place glass tube and wick into bottle. Note: The tube should barely extend above the top of the bottle.

3

Add essential blend to lamp oil.

4

Pour oil into glass bottle. Adjust glass tube and wick if necessary.

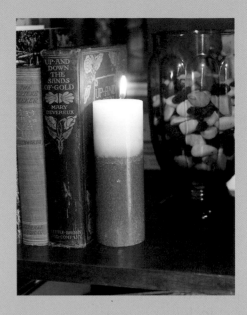

tip

Light blue lamp oil could be used to simulate the ocean.

Petitgrain blends well with:
- jasmine
- lemon
- lime
- orange

Other benefits and uses for petitgrain:
- enhances sleep
- improves memory
- relieves stress
- soothes body and mind

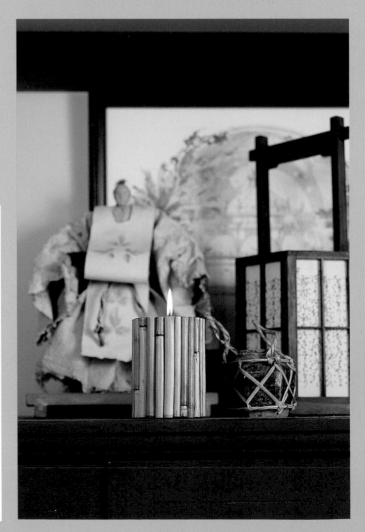

CHEERY PETITGRAIN

beach glass
clear lamp oil
decorative bottle: clear
essential oils: cedarwood, petitgrain,
    rosemary
glass tube with wick
seashells: including sea horses and
    starfish
wire cutters

Essential Blend

Cedarwood, 1 drop
Petitgrain, 3 drops
Rosemary, 1 drop

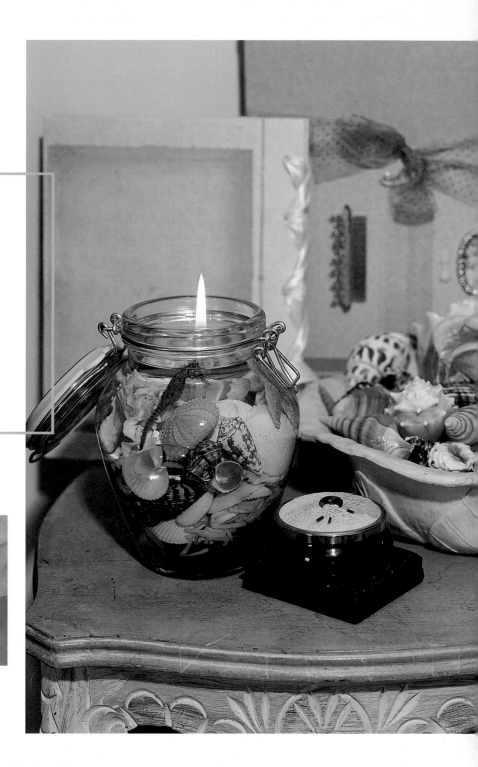

PETITGRAIN has a middle to top note with a fresh citrus fragrance that has a hint of floral. This scent is somewhat reminiscent of neroli, only lighter and less woody. Petitgrain is strengthening, especially for those who are convalescing or grieving. It brings balance back into life as well as giving a feeling of well being.

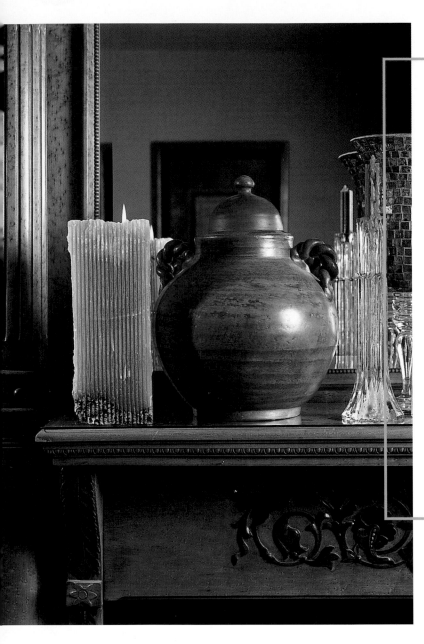

MELLOW MANDARIN

aquarium rocks: black
corrugated cardboard
double boiler
dye: orange
essential oils: clary sage, mandarin
    orange, neroli
hairpins
kitchen scale
metal pouring pot
metal skewer
mold release
mold sealer
mold: tall triangular
mold-blend wax
primed wick: square-braided
scissors
small tin container
spray vegetable oil
thermometer

Essential Blend

Clary sage, 5 drops
Mandarin orange, 13 drops
Neroli, 7 drops

MANDARIN ORANGE has a top
note with a refreshing and sweet citrus scent, which is soothing to the nerves. The sweet and delicate aroma brings joy and aids restlessness in both children and adults.

corrugated candle

1 Using double boiler, melt wax.

2 Cut corrugated cardboard to fit snugly inside of triangular mold.

3 Using mold release, lightly coat inside of mold.

4 Using spray vegetable oil, coat corrugated side of cardboard.

5 Place corrugated cardboard with corrugated side in into mold. Secure cardboard against inside edge of mold by placing hair pins through center of corrugation and over outside edge of mold.

6 Cut wick to appropriate length and thread through hole in bottom of mold and secure.

7 Place aquarium rocks 1"–2" deep in bottom of mold.

8 Pour melted wax into metal pouring pot.

9 Add dye to melted wax.

10 Add essential blend to melted wax.

11 Pour melted wax into mold until 90% full. Allow wax to set. Note: An indentation will form as wax cools, which is a design element of this candle. Excess wax may be remelted and indentation filled if desired.

12 Tip mold upside down and remove candle.

13 Remove cardboard from sides of candle. Do not worry about small bits of corrugation that may remain adhered to sides of candle, this enhances the design.

14 Trim wick at top and bottom of candle.

Mandarin orange blends well with:
> chamomile
> lemon
> sandalwood

Other benefits and uses for mandarin orange:
> antidepressant
> enhances sleep
> refreshing
> relieves stress

CEDARWOOD

has a base note with a balsamic woody fragrance. It gives strength in time of crisis and is stabilizing, grounding, and harmonizing. It brings balance to life and reminds one of their own inner strength.

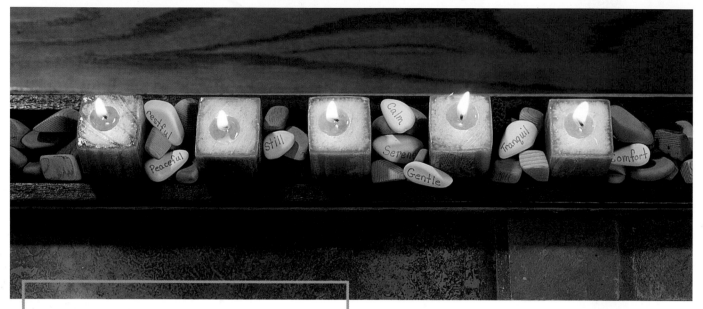

SUNNY CEDAR

double boiler
dyes: green, orange
essential oils: cedarwood, mandarin
    orange, vetiver
kitchen scale
metal pouring pot
mold: square votives (3)
mold release
mold sealer
mold-blend wax (enough to make 5
    votives)
scissors
small tin container
thermometer
wicks: paper or wire core
wick tabs (5)

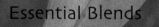

Essential Blends

Orange votives:
Cedarwood, 2 drops
Mandarin orange, 3 drops

Green votives:
Cedarwood, 2 drops
Vetiver, 2 drops

double-scented votives

1 Using double boiler, melt wax.

2 Using mold release, lightly coat inside of molds.

3 Cut wick to appropriate length and secure to wick tab. Repeat for remaining wick tabs.

4 Secure wicks to bottom of molds.

5 Pour ⅗ of melted wax into metal pouring pot.

6 Add orange dye to melted wax.

7 Add orange votive essential blend to melted wax.

8 Pour melted wax into molds until 90% full. Pour excess wax into tin container. Allow wax to set.

9 Remelt excess wax and fill indentation. Allow wax to set.

10 Tip molds upside down and remove candles.

11 Trim wicks at tops of candles.

12 Repeat Steps 2–4 for two molds.

13 Repeat Steps 5–11 with remaining wax, green dye, and green votive essential blend.

tip

Write symbolic words on decorative rocks with permanent marker.

Cedarwood blends well with:
- bergamot
- jasmine
- juniper berry
- neroli

Other benefits and uses for cedarwood:
- antidepressant
- relieves anxiety
- soothes body and mind

TOUCH

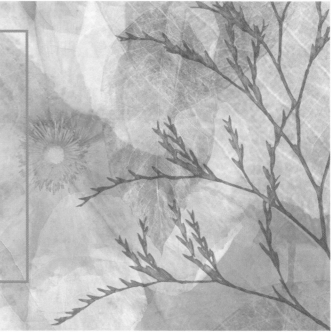

EARTH

Caring
Caution
Harmony
Home
Nurturing
Progress
Security
Stability

Touch is the most intimate, affectionate, and sometimes soothing sense. It is the one sense that humans cannot survive without. It is that which we wrap ourselves in on long cold winter nights or lightly cover ourselves with as the fireflies dance on summer evenings. It is the feeling of all that is soft and sublime. A newborn baby's cheek, a fluffy pillow almost overflowing with the finest goose down, the feel of freshly tilled soil, rich with new life. It is only a touch that can calm us, give us confidence, or guide us as we journey on our way. When you close your eyes and remember which of the senses is most memorable: how it looked? how it smelled? how it tasted? how it sounded? or how it felt?

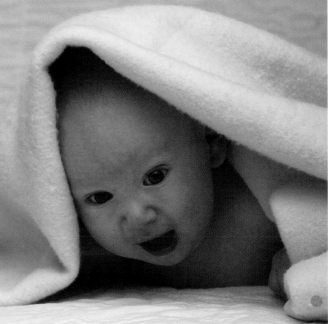

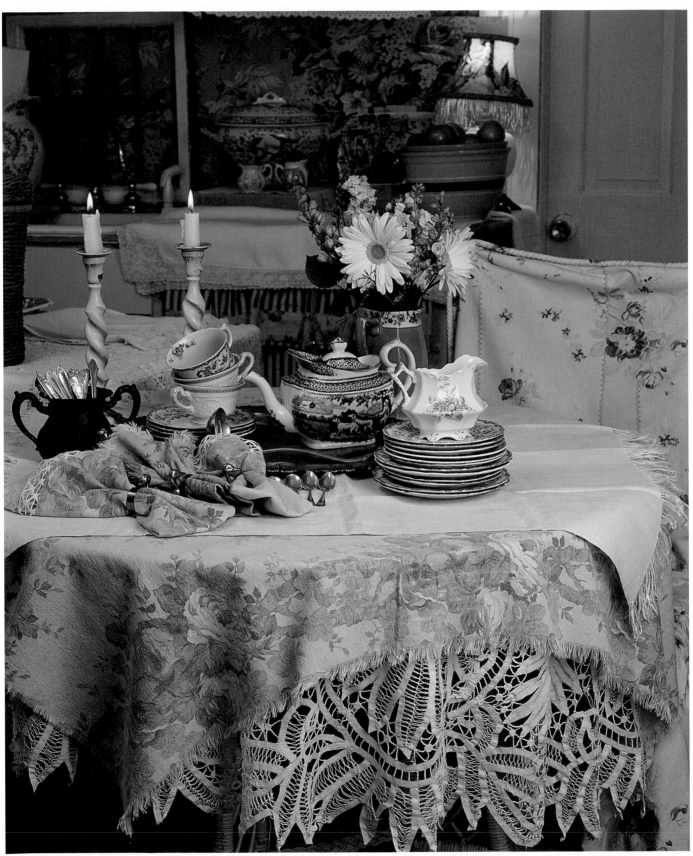

METRIC TABLE

LENGTH

metric	equivalent	imperial
1 millimetre [mm]	1 mm	0.0394 in.
1 centimetre [cm]	10 mm	0.3937 in.
1 metre [m]	100 cm	1.0936 yd.
1 kilometre[km]	1000 m	0.6214 mi.

imperial	equivalent	metric
1 inch [in.]	1 in.	2.54 cm
1 foot [ft.]	12 in.	0.3048 m
1 yard [yd.]	3 ft.	0.9144 m
1 mile [mi.]	1760 yd.	1.6093 km
1 int. nautical mi.	2025.4 yd.	1.852 km

WEIGHT

metric	equivalent	imperial
1 milligram [mg]	1 mg	0.0154 grain
1 gram [g]	1000 mg	0.0353 oz.
1 kilogram [kg]	1000 g	2.2046 lb.
1 tonne [t]	1000 kg	0.9842 ton

imperial	equivalent	metric
1 ounce [oz.]	437.5 grain	28.35 g
1 pound [lb.]	16 oz.	0.4536 kg
1 ton	20 cwt	1.016 t

VOLUME

imperial	equivalent	metric
1 teaspoon [tsp.]	5 ml	
3 tsp	1 [tbsp.]	15 ml
2 tablespoon [tbsp.]	1 fl. oz.	30 ml
1 cup	8 fl. oz.	0.24 litre [l]
2 cups	1 pint [pt.]	0.47 l
4 cups	1 quart [qt.]	0.95 l
4 qts.	1 gallon [gal.]	3.8 l
16 tbsp.	1 cup	0.24 l

imperial	UK equivalent	metric
1 fluid ounce [fl. oz.]	1.0408 UK fl. oz.	29.574 ml
1 pt.	0.8327 UK pt.	0.4731 l
1 gal.	0.8327 UK gal.	3.7854 l

TEMPERATURE CONVERSION EQUATIONS
Degrees Farenheit (°F) to degrees Celsius (°C)

°F to °C	=	(°F – 32) × 5/9
°C to °F	=	(°C × 9/5) + 32

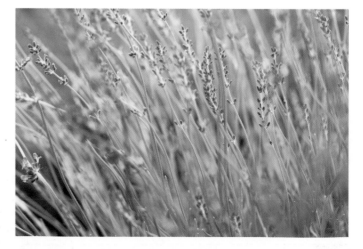

INDEX